SWIMMING FOR FITNESS AND FUN

SWIMMING FOR FITNESS AND FUN

John Learmouth

DAVID & CHARLES
NEWTON ABBOT . LONDON
NORTH POMFRET (VT) . VANCOUVER

ISBN 0 7153 71827

Library of Congress Catalog Card Number
76-8703

Set in 11 on 13pt. Times
and printed in Great Britain
by Redwood Burn   Trowbridge and Esher
for David & Charles (Publishers) Limited
Brunel House Newton Abbot Devon

Published in the United States of America
by David & Charles Inc
North Pomfret   Vermont 05053   USA

Published in Canada
by Douglas David & Charles Limited
1875 Welch Street North Vancouver   BC

Contents

List of Illustrations

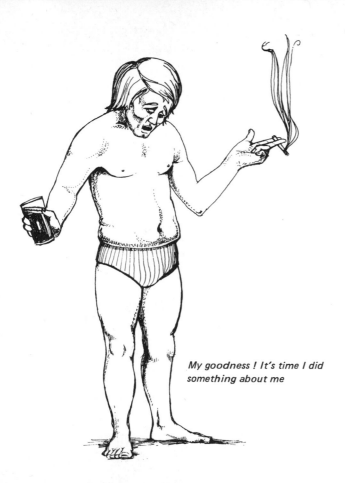

My goodness! It's time I did something about me

1 Swimming and Health

By way of an introduction, I thought you might be interested in some recent history. It is all about Mike, the chap pictured opposite, although I suppose it might be about any one of thousands of people. Although he doesn't like very much to admit it, he's on the wrong side of thirty-five – and he smokes too much. He drinks a bit, as well; he doesn't eat any too wisely and, of course, he works under continual pressure – but then, who doesn't, these days? He's also carrying a bit too much weight, and, at the back of his mind, he worries about all this and its effect on his health. He tells me that his way of life, the very manner in which he earns his daily bread, is the main contributory factor to all of this, and for this reason he has never been very success-ful in his periodic attempts to cut down on his various excesses. What he would like to do, so he says, is to undertake some form of regular exercise which is fun to take part in, which is safe – in terms of the avoidance of the possibility of overstrain – and which will help to counteract the adverse effects of his way of life.

Mike poured all this out to me at a party one evening. I asked him if he could swim, and he admitted that it was an awfully long time since he had done so. Yet for a person in his situation, swimming is the ideal exercise. Paradoxically, in the early stages, the worse you are at it, the better the physical benefits, because a bad swimmer has to put a lot more physical effort into struggling across a width than a good one does into swimming a length or two. Seemingly unimpressed Mike wanted to know, 'Why swimming?'. I then gave him the following list of reasons, both day-to-day practical and in terms of an improvement in health:

Swimming can be done almost entirely at times of your own choosing. Most swimming pools are open from early in the morning until late in the evening. Most of us can find half an hour at some time during this period. You don't need a partner, an opponent, or a team in order to take part, which means that you can go at times of your own choosing and not be dependent upon someone else's convenience.

Swimming is an inexpensive pastime. Admission charges are very reasonable, and there is no expensive equipment to buy.

It is an all-the-year-round pastime – regardless of season or weather.

Age is no barrier in recreational swimming. It is therefore the ideal family recreation, in which parents and children (and grandparents if they wish) may take part with equal success and enjoyment.

There is an increasing availability of facilities, many in delightful surroundings at sports and leisure centres.

Swimming is a most useful skill insofar as it contributes to one's own safety and to that of others, and it is a pre-requisite for admission to other water sports.

There is an increasing involvement by parents in their children's recreation. Anything you are able to do to help your children to learn to swim must be beneficial – provided that you know what you are doing! This extends from mother and baby groups up to the point where the child is being taught to swim properly.

So far as physical health is concerned, I continued, warming to my subject, swimming is just about the perfect form of exercise for people of all ages. Whenever the average adult takes up some form of physical recreation, having done very little physically for some time, there is always the danger that he may overdo it, and finish up by doing himself more harm than good. When this happens, it is almost always the result of being forced to play at a pace dictated by an opponent, a partner, or a book of rules. One of the beauties of recreational swimming is that you can do it at your own pace, and thus minimise the possibility of overstrain. Any increase in effort to effect improvements in physical efficiency can be carefully graduated, to allow the bodily systems to 'gear up' gradually rather than all at once.

The heart, of course, is just a rather specialised muscle, and shares most of its characteristics with all the other muscles in the body. One of these characteristics is that its efficiency may be improved through regular exercise. It will not increase in size as a result of exercise, unlike the biceps, for example, but it will certainly become stronger and more efficient. The same is true of the muscles which are concerned with breathing.

There is also the quite interesting fact that, when the human body is in the normal upright position, most of the blood which is returning to the heart for recircula-tion has to travel almost vertically uphill. And this, mark you, after having lost most of the pumping force of the heart – this was used up on the outward journey. The physical effects of this contribute to many circulatory problems. Swimming is fairly unique in that the exercise is carried out with the body in a horizontal position, and there is thus little or no gravitational opposition to the blood returning to the heart. It is in recognition of this that competitive swimmers, at the end of a hard race, very seldom stand erect immediatly. They rather tend to push off again, usually on the back, and gently swim up the pool and back before standing upright, thus avoiding giving the additional strain of gravity to a heart which has been working very hard. So, in terms of circulation, swimming is probably the safest form of physical recreation.

Another interesting and physically beneficial facet of swimming which is obtained without conscious effort on the part of the swimmer is brought about by the fact that the trunk is immersed in water. In this situation the respiratory mechanism has to work against the resistance of water pressure, which is greater than the air pressure which is the normal resistance. The additional effort involved, although generally unnoticed by the swimmer, strengthens the respiratory muscles and generally makes everyday breathing more efficient.

If a person is trying to improve his swimming, and by doing so to improve his general bodily fitness, the improvement in both can be easily measured. The realisation that improvements are taking place gives a tremendous psychological incentive to keep at it. In swimming technique, the progress is self-evident, even if only because swimming becomes a bit easier to do. In terms of fitness, simple pulse-rate checks, made while in the water and at other times, soon show (by a reduction in pulse rate) that the circulation is becoming more efficient.

Having listened to all of this, Mike decided to give it a go. He has not been at it all that long, but he is delighted with the results, thus far. He has become very pulse- and breathing-conscious, and he has lately persuaded himself not to smoke for one hour before going to the pool and for one hour after he comes out. He says that, having given his lungs a good airing, he wants to delay coking them up again. He is also very proud of the fact that his resting pulse-rate is down to slightly below normal. What is happening to Mike, of course, is that when he decided to take up swimming on a regular basis, he adopted a more positive attitude toward his health, and since he is now making the effort to go to the baths practically every day, he is psychologically able to think in terms of making additional contributions to his physical well-being, such as cutting down on his smoking.

He says he finds it most relaxing, mentally as well as physically, and that he is marvellously refreshed by his daily swim, even although he is still at the stage where he is aware of having made a physical effort when he gets out of the water. On the debit side, his jackets are beginning to feel a little tight about the shoulders, and his trousers a little loose around the waist. He's still far from looking like Adonis, mind you, but he is looking better than he did.

That evening, when he first put his problem into words, I offered to write him a set of programmes, which were designed to improve his swimming. By working through them, he would gain the physical benefits he wanted. The better he was able to swim, the more he would enjoy it. The more he enjoyed it, the more often he would swim – and the more often he swam the fitter he would become. A beneficial circle, rather than the more usual vicious one.

Since Mike is reasonably intelligent, it was obvious that he would react better to the instructions in his programme if he understood why he was being asked to do certain things. Hence the occasional digression in and among the techniques and the descriptions of exercises. Here I have reproduced all Mike's programmes for the various techniques and strokes in the following chapters. Perhaps you'd like to have a go?

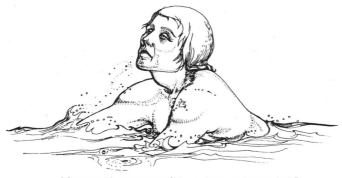

Of course I'm water confident - I can swim can't I ?

2   The Basics

Good swimming is impossible without water confidence. It is a sad fact that very many people, who are in fact able to swim, do so quite badly because they lack the confidence to adopt the position in the water that the stroke demands. This almost always means that they are not happy to swim with their faces submerged throughout most of the stroke cycle. Where this applies to a child, one is dealing with a situation of conscious fear – the child will readily admit that he is frightened to have his face submerged because the water might go up his nose, or in his mouth, or in his eyes or ears.

The average adult may still have this fear, but it is largely subconscious. He has little awareness of being actually frightened by the situation, and would maintain that he swims in this particular way because he prefers to do so. His attempts to swim, say, Crawl, are doomed to failure because he prefers to swim with his head above the surface. When you come to Chapter 4 you will see why. But it still comes down to a matter of lack of water confidence, whether consciously admitted or not. Fortunately, the great majority of adults are able to acquire this confidence through various exercises, provided that they understand why it is necessary to do them.

The first important factor to understand is human flotation. The average adult has a specific gravity of around 0.99. Without being technical this effectively means that a human body will float, but with 99 per cent of its mass below the surface and only about 1 per cent above. What we gather from this is that one swims through water, not on it. Factor number two is that the legs, having large bones and a lot of muscle, are the densest part of this fairly dense mass, and are therefore always trying to sink, and unless one does something positive to stop it happening, sink they will! Thus, in fresh water, the natural floating position of the human body is – the legs having obeyed the natural laws – the whole body floating with 99 per cent of its mass submerged. I would like you to prove this to your own satisfaction, so the first activity is this:

Hang on to the rail at a point in the pool where the water is three to six inches deeper than your own height.

Take a deep breath and hold it, and press the air hard against your tightly closed lips. It is impossible for water to enter either mouth or nose as long as you keep pressing the air against your lips.

Let go of the rail and put your arms by your side.

This is what will happen – and forewarned is forearmed. As soon as you release the rail you will sink to the bottom. Alright, hold your nose if you must, but do get round to doing it without. What I told you about the deep breath is true! When your feet touch bottom, do not push off, but just allow yourself to float back to the surface. You will, I promise you. As your head clears the surface, however, you will start to sink again, but you will not go so deep this time before you start to rise again. This up-down, up-down, will happen two or three times, and you will finally come to rest in your natural flotation position, which will be as shown in Fig 1, probably with your mouth just below the surface. Your buoyancy has been enhanced by the fact that you have a lungful of air, of which more later.

It may be that you will have to do this quite a few times before you are able to hold your breath for long enough to get to the point where your are vertically

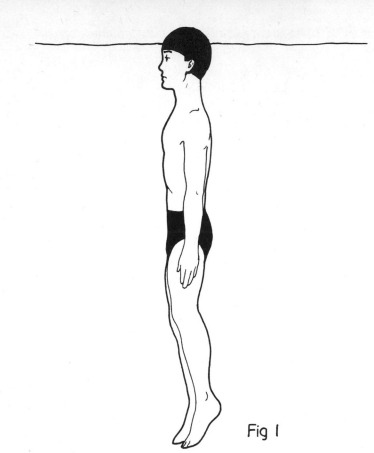

Fig 1

floating, quite motionless; but this is no bad thing, as you are learning a lot about your own flotation, and gaining genuine water-confidence and improving your general watermanship all the time.

Mike was lucky when he was going through this, since he was carrying a little excess weight. Fat is the only tissue in the human body which will float, and the more you have, the lower your body's specific gravity, and the more of your mass will be above the surface. This is why women tend to float higher than men, since their bodies contain a higher proportion of fatty tissue.

You will find that you can hold the vertical floating position and breathe as well, by slowly tilting your head back until your mouth is clear of the surface, and doing a fast, shallow breathing action through the mouth. This type of breathing action allows inhalation and exhalation to take place while keeping the lungs fairly full of air. A long, full exhalation would blow most of the air out of the lungs and you would lose a lot of your buoyancy.

As a second activity, I'd like you to prove this. In the same starting position as before, blow out as much air as you can and, pressing the remaining air against your tightly closed lips to stop water coming in, release the rail as you did last time. You will notice that you do not rise to the surface as quickly as before, and when you finally come to rest you will be much lower in the water – with the top of your head just breaking, or even just below, the surface. Some people, especially tall, slim men, will not float back to the surface at all, until they push themselves up with their feet. I am one of the latter type, and can quite happily sit or lie on the bottom of the pool. It's quite fun, if you can do it.

When you have done these exercises a few times, you should be convinced that:

Provided you apply sufficient internal air pressure to the inside of your compressed lips, and thus automatically to the nasal passages, no water can possibly enter your mouth or nose, no matter how far you are beneath the surface of a swimming pool. It's a simple matter of causing your internal air pressure to become greater than the water pressure at the possible points of entry.

Your natural flotation position has about 99 per cent of your body mass below the surface without lungs filled with air. If your lungs are full you can float slightly higher. The corollary to this is that if you try to get more than the 1 per cent, give or take a little, above the surface, you will sink below the surface before the

laws of hydrostatics come into play to return you to your proper flotation position. Remember what happened when you started doing this. Holding the rail, you had the whole of your head and most of your forearms above the surface – maybe 7 or 8 per cent of your mass. As soon as you released the rail the natural laws took over and down you went. I'd like you to remember this later, when we get on to the effects of swimming with the head above the surface.

Motion helps to overcome this unfortunate effect of the high specific gravity of the human body. As Newton stated (more or less) in his first law, once a body has been set in motion it will continue on a constant course and at a constant speed until some other force intervenes. If you push yourself off from the side of the pool, in a horizontal position, you will glide across the pool. The body has been set in motion, and would theoretically now go on for ever but for the other forces. The first of these is the friction between your body's surface and the water itself, which slows your progress fairly quickly. As you lose your speed, the laws of flotation take over and your legs start to sink. If you are in water which is sufficiently deep, you will finish up in the vertical position with half your head above the surface,

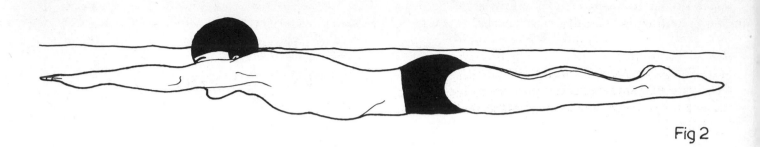

Fig 2

just as you did before. It does prove, however, that all the time the body is in motion it enjoys considerably more buoyancy.

This business of gliding in the horizontal position (*See Fig 2*) is the absolute foundation of good swimming. If you can glide well, you can learn to swim well. If you cannot, you will certainly never swim Crawl, and you will make the swimming of other strokes much harder work for yourself.

Can we have a go at it, then?

Stand, facing the rail and about five feet from it, in waist to chest depth. Stretch your arms out ahead of you, palms downward, and lock the thumbs one over the other.

Bend at the knees until your shoulders are completely submerged.

Take a deep breath, compress your lips, drop your head until your ears are between your upper arms, and push yourself through (not over, but through) the water to the rail.

Grasp the rail and stand up, and don't wipe your face with your hands – let it drip! You've got to get used to water on your face – after all, there is no known stroke which has an arm action which goes, *pull, wipe, pull, wipe*. This action is called 'push and glide' and I shall be constantly referring to it. It is very important.

I'd like you to repeat the push and glide to the rail many

times, trying to increase your distance, and paying particular attention to the following points:

Try to get your arms, shoulders and head below the surface as you push off. Remember, you're trying to glide through the water. You achieve this by a deeper bend of the knees as your are 'gathering' to push.

As soon as your feet leave the pool bottom, get your body into the longest, thinnest position possible. A tight thumb-lock, arms stretched hard, legs stretched hard, knees and ankles pressed together and feet pointed. This is a matter of simple streamlining, to minimise water resistance.

If you're not already doing so, try opening your eyes as you glide. This is a fairly essential point of water confidence, and you've got to get around to it, even if it means wearing a pair of swimming goggles in your early stages if your eyes are very sensitive to chlorinated water.

I'd like you to take especial note, at this point, of the motions you go through in the process of standing up when you have reached the rail. Apart from the little pull on the rail, these are exactly the same motions that you go through when you want to stand from the

horizontal position and there is no rail to grasp, eg halfway across the width. What you are doing is the following sequence of movements (*See Fig 3*):

Pull down with your hands.

Bend your knees and lift them toward the chest.

Lift up your face until it is well clear of the water.

Try a few glides into the rail, and note how this is, in fact, the way in which you have been regaining your feet. Say to yourself, as you do it, 'Pull down, head up, knees up.'

Now try to regain your feet just before you get to the rail. The only action that is in any way different from what you have been doing is that, as you pull down, you keep your arms straight, so that they go straight down in their stretched position. Don't pull too vigorously or too quickly, just a smooth easy pull. Now that you're confident that you can regain your feet from the glide position, without needing a rail to grab, we'll try pushing and gliding from the wall and across the pool, but before we set off there is a modification to the breathing technique that we must introduce. It's called the 'explosive' technique, and is widely used

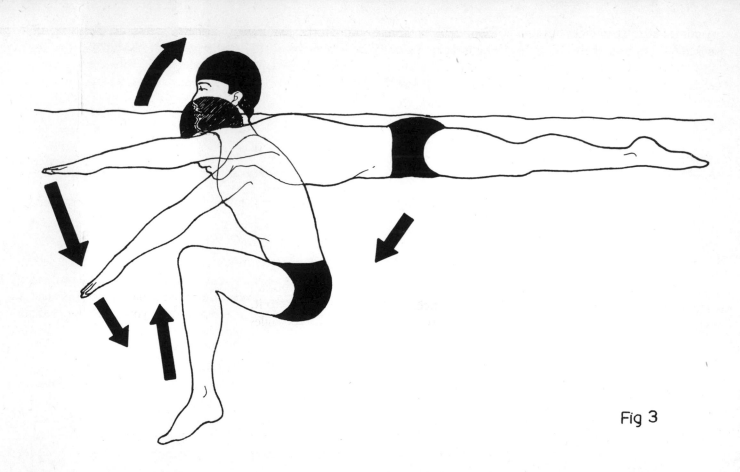

Fig 3

by competitive swimmers but not so frequently by those seeking to improve their swimming; which seems a great pity, since the latter category needs its benefits as much as, and probably more than, the former. It's nothing very complicated. All you have to do is exhale first, then inhale; both through the mouth. You can practise this anywhere.

First, you forcibly and quickly blow the air out through your pursed lips. It is an 'explosive' action, and makes a marked 'pff' sound. Immediately following the blowing out you inhale, virtually sucking the air in through the still-pursed lips, and as soon as you have drawn the air in you clamp your lips together tightly. When you first begin to breathe this way, it will be a matter of *out-in*, *out-in*, but as you get used to it the two actions will merge into one: *outin*, *outin*.

Looking back over what you have already done, the advantages of this method of breathing are probably obvious. First, we know that a lungful of air considerably enhances buoyancy. Using this technique, there is only a split second when the lungs are not full, whereas with the traditional method of breathing you inhale and then immediately start dribbling the air out, losing buoyancy all the time you are doing so. Second, knowing that only 1 per cent of the body is going to be above the surface, we realise that the mouth is never going to be very much above the surface. In this situation, a forcible exhalation before inhaling will blow away any water that may be in the vicinity of the lips. This way, it does not get sucked in with the air. From this point on, we'll do everything using this explosive breathing technique:

Stand, back to the wall, arms stretched, thumbs locked together, knees bent and shoulders under the water. (Through it, not on it; remember?)

Put one foot against the wall, take a deep breath (out, in) and drop your head until your ears are touching your upper arms.

Put the other foot against the wall, letting the head sink below the surface, and push.

Hold the glide (long thin position, everything stretched) until you lose speed and almost stop. Pull down, knees up, head up, and there you are, standing.

Keep practising this until you can shoot through the water like an arrow, long thin and relaxed, for eight or so metres.

You just cannot practise this one too much. The most vital thing in swimming is a correct body position, and the push and glide position is perfection. Variations of the push and glide which are well worth trying, because they are fun to do and because they will teach you watermanship skills which will be useful later, are:

Push and glide to the pool bottom. When you push off, lower your head and arms to direct your glide downward instead of forward. Hold the long stretched position, and as your hands touch bottom, point them up toward the surface, and you will glide up to the surface.

A variation on this is to push and glide to the bottom, and then to start working the legs up and down – as for Crawl – and, still in the stretched position, complete the width underwater. To do this it is essential that you keep your eyes open, otherwise you are liable to collide with other people's legs or finish up by ramming into the wall. (At this point in the game a pair of flippers is a most useful piece of equipment, but do inquire of the baths manager whether their use is permitted before committing yourself to the expense of buying. If you do buy, however, get the best you can afford. Avoid flippers which are secured by a strap around the heel;

the straps break, they get lost, and even when they are new they are none too secure on the feet. Go for a pair which are like an extended shoe, where the whole foot is in the flipper. The increase in leg propulsion obtained from flippers makes swimming much easier and more fun to do, and is invaluable when you are trying to improve the Crawl strokes.)

Back push and glide. This is, as its name suggests, nothing more than the push and glide done on the back. Stand facing the rail and holding it with your hands spaced about shoulder-width apart. Lift both feet about a foot up the wall. Take a deep breath, compress the lips, and with a steady rather than an explosive effort push with the feet, release the rail, and stretch out, with the hands by the sides. Adopt the long, stretched body position (except that the arms are by the sides) and glide. The head should be on its natural line with the body, ie looking straight up at the ceiling. To regain the standing position from back push and glide, the actions are the same as before – pull down, knees up, head up.

A more advanced method of doing back push and glide involves the same starting position and take-off, but instead of pulling the arms in to the side you should throw them back beyond the head as far as they will go and lock the thumbs together when they get there. Thus you are in the same position as for front push and glide, but on the back instead of the front.

This is an almost identical action to that of a Back Crawl racing start and, in order to get the arms clear of the water so that they may be thrown back, it is necessary to lift yourself higher up the wall before driving back. This is one of the very, very few actions in swimming where a deliberate attempt is made to get part of the body going over the water, rather than through it.

Once you are satisfied that you are quite happy on the push and glide and all its variations, there is one more thing I'd like you to do, as a flotation and confidence exercise. This is the 'mushroom float', and this is a true measure of your buoyancy (*See Fig 4*):

Stand in waist- to chest-depth water. Take a deep breath and compress the lips.

Lift the knees to the chest, grasp the knees with the hands and pull them in to the chest. Push your chin down in to your chest – and float. The only part of your body which will be above the surface will be a small area of your back – a true 1 per cent of your body mass.

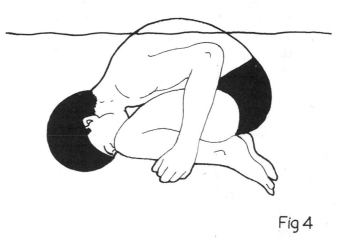

Fig 4

Once you have done this a few times, it is quite interesting to get into the mushroom float position, and then blow out as much air as you can, and see how much further down you will go. This indicates to what extent your buoyancy is due to the presence of air in the lungs, and how much is due to natural flotation. Those with a bodily specific gravity which is higher than 1.00, having expelled the air, will slowly sink to the bottom, but this is a relatively rare occurrence in adults.

Having done all of these basic activities, you are

21

ready to go on to the strokes themselves, but even while you are working at the strokes you should devote a little time to these basic exercises, particularly the push and glide. There are many factors which go together to make up a good swimming stroke, but the most important of these is body position. If body position is correct it is possible for the other factors to come right, but if the body position is not right then nothing else can happen correctly. The position you are in when doing a good push and glide is the ideal body-position for swimming. When performing a stroke, it is not always possible to maintain this position, but good swimming is really all about trying to do so. I started this chapter by advancing the proposition that, with adults, understanding of what is involved is essential to success. Think about body position, whatever you are doing. Play about with these basic exercises. Try doing them with a raised head, with a lowered head and with limbs in different positions. Observe what happens as a result of the variations, and work out the reason.

Merely for the sake of having them in a convenient list, now that you know why you are doing them and what to expect, here again are the practices I'd like you to go through:

1 Flotation tests. Vertical floating from the rail, with air, with 'flutter' breathing, and without air.

2 Push and glide. To the rail, and regaining the feet.

3 Explosive breathing.

4 Push and glide. From the rail, to the bottom, and to swim underwater.

5 Back push and glide.

6 Mushroom float.

Before leaving these basic exercises it should be said that, if anyone is uncertain of his ability to start any of them happily, a polystyrene float is a most useful aid for the push and glide practices. They are cheap to buy, and are not frowned upon in swimming pools. Held in both hands in the push and glide position, and held on the chest when on the back, they provide that extra buoyancy which none of us really needs, but with which many of us feel a great deal happier.

One last fact that I would like you to appreciate before going on to the various strokes is that in all of them arm actions play havoc with the ideal body position which we've worked so hard to perfect. It is all a matter of Newton's Third Law of Motion – for every action there will be an equal and opposite reaction. Thus – and think of any swimming arm-action you like – if an arm moves downward through water, the body is propelled upward. If it moves backward, the body will be propelled forward. If we could so organise swimming strokes so that all arm actions were pure backward movements, we would get pure forward propulsion and few problems with body position. As things are, there are of necessity downward, upward, outward and inward components in arm actions, and these bring inevitable opposite reactions in body position. If the reaction is upward to the extent that the entire head and perhaps even the top of the shoulders are lifted clear of the water, which happens in Breast Stroke, the legs will start to sink, and the horizontal body position will be lost.

Fortunately leg actions, whether markedly propulsive or not, constantly correct the body position, mainly by pushing the legs up toward the surface all the time, thus maintaining the horizontal.

We have said that good swimming is all about body position. Equally, body position is all about efficient leg actions, and for this reason every swimming stroke must be learned in the same way, ie push and glide into leg action. There is absolutely no point in going on to full stroke until the leg action is efficient and automatic.

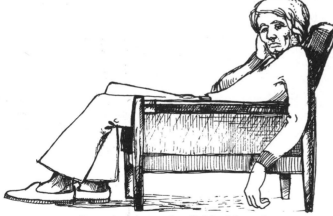

I can relax my muscles all right, It's getting some tension into them that's my problem

3   The Swimming Session

The same principles that apply to a session undertaken by a competitive swimmer apply to anyone who is undertaking exercise on a structured basis. Every session should start with a five-minute 'warm-up', to gear up the bodily systems to cope with the more than ordinary demands that are going to be made upon them. Similarly, at the end of the session there should be a five-minute 'ease-down' to return the systems gradually to a situation of normality. You would not think of switching off your car engine while it was racing at full revs; you let it run down to tickover before switching off. The same applies to the human body.

Warm-up

This should consist of reasonably gentle activities, the precise nature of which will depend upon the stage you have reached in swimming proficiency. For the swimmer who is working on the basics, the warm-up could well consist of going through the flotation and confidence exercises, together with some work on push and glide. The more competent swimmer who is working on stroke improvement would probably warm up on push and glide, gentle legs-only exercises and perhaps full stroke, using a stroke he can swim reasonably well. The warm-up period may also be used to revise activities previously done, but, whatever form it takes, it should last for a full five minutes.

Ease-down

This, too, should last for a full five minutes. For the swimmer who is on the basics the content might well be the same as for the warm-up. I like to see underwater activities as part of an ease-down session, because the puffing and blowing that tends to result gets rid of the carbon dioxide which has built up in the body as a result of the more severe exercise recently undertaken. The beginner could include things like push and glide to the pool bottom, while the more advanced could undertake some underwater swimming for a given distance. Do not set yourself stiff targets. Remember that you are easing down. Water tricks, like hand-standing in the water or the early diving exercises shown, are also good to include. Floating activities are useful, in that they give you something positive to do while not being very physically demanding.

When you finally leave the water, have a hot shower. If you are able, reduce the temperature to blood heat, which will feel cool but not cold, for half a minute or so before leaving the shower.

Relaxation

As soon as other people know that you have taken up swimming, they will start giving you advice, all of which, even though perhaps not appropriate, is very well meant. As Damon Runyon would have it, it's no better than five to four that you will be advised to relax. Should this happen, it is important that you know what relaxation, in swimming, is about. Basically, every swimmer at any level of performance must have an acceptable level of general relaxation (loose and floppy). This assists flotation, it enables you to let the water carry you instead of fighting it all the time and, above all, it enables you to make the necessary movements in a smooth and graceful manner, which is absolutely essential to good swimming. I cannot think of any swimming stroke which, swum well, does not look easy and graceful, even lazy, except for Dolphin Butterfly, and even that, swum slowly, looks attractive. The achievement of general relaxation is almost entirely a matter of water confidence, so if anyone tells you to relax in the early stages, what he really means is, 'Be confident'.

Having achieved general relaxation, through water confidence, every swimmer has the need of specific relaxation, which is a much more sophisticated business. This is the somewhat negative art of stopping a group of muscles which are not supposed to be working from preventing the muscles which are supposed to be working from doing their job efficiently. This is something for the advanced swimmer to worry about, and can only be achieved to its fullest possible extent by miles and miles of swimming, coupled with a good working knowledge of skeletal and muscular anatomy. By the time you get to swimming lengths, you will have achieved, without knowing you've done so, sufficient specific relaxation to do all you wish to do.

4 The Crawl

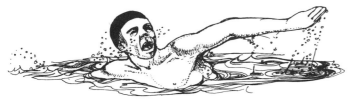

My Crawl Stroke's fine, it's just that I can't do it and breathe as well

A short – and therefore somewhat oversimplified – way of describing functions in Crawl could read: 'The arms propel, and in doing so, ruin the body position. The legs therefore have to work at three times the speed of the arms to try to correct and maintain a reasonable body position, since without it, breathing is impossible.'

Any normal person can perform a functionally acceptable Crawl arm-action, almost without tuition, once he has seen it done. Most people can perform a reasonable leg action – in isolation. What most people cannot do is perform the leg action reasonably when they have to do it at the same time as the arm action, and in a different rhythmic beat. The arms are working in a 1, 2 : 1, 2, rhythm, while at the same time the legs are working in a 1, 2, 3, 4, 5, 6 : 1, 2, 3, 4, 5, 6 rhythm. This demands a complete disassociation of timing very much like the rhythmic difference between the right and left hands when playing boogie-woogie on a piano. If you cannot do this, you cannot maintain the near-horizontal body position necessary to create the right hydrostatic conditions which make breathing possible.

So you will appreciate that the foundation of a good Crawl is a sound leg-action. We must therefore get this right before we try to do anything else. Fortunately, there are sufficient variations of practices to prevent boredom. When I am training swimming teachers, I always make the point that at the moment when you start your pupil practising for Crawl leg-action, he has got about two thousand widths of 'legs only' swimming ahead of him before it becomes anything near to the habit action we are after. The only chance of avoiding boredom and of maintaining interest lies in continual variation in the way the practices are done. The pupil has got to keep doing the same thing – the good teacher can find many different ways in which he can do it.

The first exercise can be done almost anywhere – in the water, at the office, providing nobody is watching, or at home:

Stretch both legs (no bend at the knee) and point the toes. Move the legs alternately up and down, so that each foot is travelling about fifteen inches on each movement. The movement comes from the hip joint, and there is no movement in the knee joint whatsoever. The whole thing is done with straight legs. While you are doing it, count the six-beat rhythm *1,2,3,4,5,6, 1,2,3,4,5,6* . . . You have got to fix this rhythm in your mind to an extent that every time, for evermore, that you start to do this action, your mind will be chanting the rhythm for you.

At the swimming pool, this is done by lying horizontally on the water in the push and glide position with the face in the water, holding the rail. When you need to breathe, turn the head sideways and lift it slightly until the mouth is clear of the water, and use the explosive breathing technique. Having inhaled, return the head to its proper position with the face in the water. This practice may also be usefully done when either sitting in a chair or, better still, lying on your back on the floor. The fact that you are facing upward, when in the stroke you would be facing downward, does not matter at all. We are trying to establish a pattern of movement done to a fixed rhythm, and whether this is practised on front, back or side, the effect will be the same. In the sitting position, and more so in the lying position, this is a strong abdominal exercise, and will tend to start to flatten any bulge at the waistline. Once this pattern is established, the next exercise is done as follows:

Stand with the back to the rail. Push and glide. As you achieve the horizontal position in the water, start the legs working while maintaining the long stretched position. The arms extended ahead of you act as a balancing agent and maintain the streamlining which is necessary to minimise the resistance to your forward movement.

When you need to breathe, stop and stand up. Please, no attempts to breathe while in the push and glide position – it cannot be done without raising the head, and if you start raising your head at this stage it will be very difficult to break the habit pattern when we want to start breathing while swimming the full stroke. When we get on to breathing, you'll see why this is so, but at the moment please take my word for it!

With proper breath control, you should be able to manage the width of the average pool without needing another breath, especially if you let your push and glide do its work and get you halfway across before you start the legs going. As you progress with this exercise, I'd like you to think about relaxing at the knee and ankle, ie holding the leg straight but not stiff. In order to obtain forward propulsion, the ankles must be loose. Indeed, when swimming with your legs only, at first, you may find that you either make no forward progress or that you even go backwards. If this happens, it is due to the ankle joint being rigidly fixed. This straight but not stiff posture of the leg is not an easy thing to obtain, but if you think about it while you are doing it it will come with practice.

Repeat this exercise on the back. The advantage of this is that you can see what your legs are doing. If your knees come out of the water, your legs are bent. Straighten them. Back push and glide; when you are horizontal, start the legs going. No breathing problems here.

In all leg-action exercises, make sure that no part of the leg or foot comes out of the water. Propulsion is obtained when some part of the body is pushing against the water, so anything that is done out of the water is just wasted effort. A pair of flippers is invaluable in the early stages. With these on your feet, you really get the 'feel' of propulsion, not only in that you are going through the water fairly quickly but, more important, in that you can feel the foot action which is causing the propulsion to happen. The leverage of the flipper causes the ankle to work correctly, whether it wants to or not.

Try the same exercise under water. In the same way as you did for your push and glide practices, push off from the side, aiming yourself at the bottom of the pool. As soon as you are totally submerged, get the legs going, while keeping the arms extended ahead of you. Do not, however, attempt this while wearing flippers, unless you are fully confident of your ability to see while under water. Flippers propel you at quite a speed, underwater, and unless you are able to see where you are going you may collide with someone else or with the pool wall, which could be quite serious.

No matter how accustomed to the leg action you are now becoming, keep counting the rhythm, *1,2,3,4,5,6 : 1,2,3,4,5,6*, and so on. We've got to create a permanent habit pattern. It is the leg action which maintains the near-horizontal body position. Remember that the legs, left to their own devices, will sink and get you into an eventual vertical position. To swim a proper and co-ordinated Crawl, the body position must be nearly horizontal, and this, above all, is what a good leg action will do for you, making all the other aspects of the stroke possible.

When you begin to feel that your legs are working as they should, try giving yourself some resistance for the legs to work against. The ideal resistance is a polystyrene float, held upright, when you are doing leg practice in the push and glide position. If you haven't got a float, the hands held in the same position will provide a good resistance. (*See Fig 5.*) This resistance is caused by the fact that you have abandoned your streamlined position and are causing your hands, or the float, to push a pile of water ahead of you. Just like pushing a loaded wheelbarrow when walking, this makes forward motion that bit harder. I want you to remember this business about pushing the pile of water ahead of you, because it is this fact of hydrodynamics which is responsible for allowing breathing to take place when swimming Crawl. More of that later.

Now that you are reasonably used to moving in the push and glide position with the legs kicking, I would like you to think about your legs in terms of relaxation. I want them straight but not rigid. The knee joint has to be held tightly enough to keep the leg basically straight, but with enough relaxation to allow it to bend very slightly against the water resistance to the downward action. At the bottom of the down kick it must be straightened immediately, so that the upward kick is done with a perfectly straight leg. This, done properly,

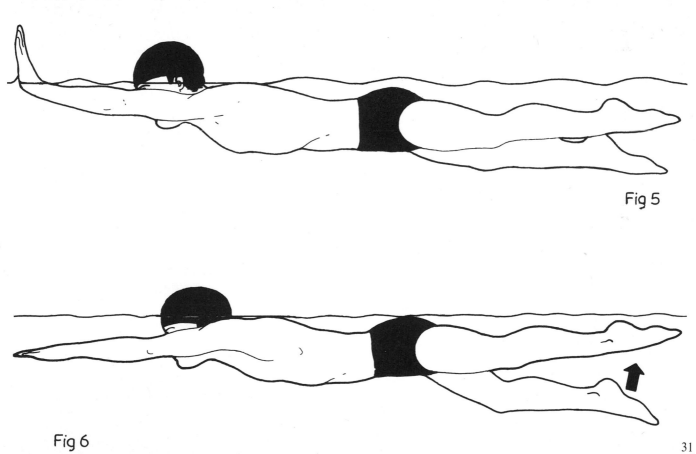

Fig 5

Fig 6

31

results in a whip-like upward action. (*See Fig 6.*) The ankle joint, meanwhile, can be as loose and floppy as you can get it. The floppier the better. The larger the range of movement in the ankle joint, the better the propulsion.

The leg-action exercises may be summarised as follows:

1 Lying at the rail; lying on your back on the carpet; sitting in a chair. (Leg action to a six-beat rhythm.)

2 Push and glide, adding leg action.

3 Back push and glide, adding leg action.

4 Push and glide to the pool bottom, adding leg action.

5 Legs only swimming, against resistance.

Arm action

I have always maintained that it is not necessary to teach anyone the Crawl arm-action. In my view and experience it is so simple that once someone has seen it done, he can copy it reasonably efficiently. All he then needs is correction on minor points of technique. Neither have I ever seen an effective arms-only exercise which is suitable for the learner or improver. Any arm-action practice which is carried out with the feet on the bottom of the pool is being carried out with the arms at the wrong angle to the trunk and, as often as not, brings sets of muscles into play which are not used, or are used differently, when the stroke as a whole is being performed. Thus a wrong habit-pattern is being formed. It is impossible while bending at the hip, as one does when performing any standing exercise, to attain a trunk posture which will allow the arms to reproduce the actual swimming action. In addition to this, the arms enter and leave the water in the wrong relative places. The arm action is best practised in a whole-stroke situation. Everything we do from now on, until we get on to breathing, must be done with held breath and the face in the water. If, while doing the exercises, you get absolutely desperate for air, then stop, stand up, breathe, and start again. Please, please, no attempts to breathe while on the move – not for a little while, anyway.

Push and glide from the side. Get the legs going and keep going, legs only, for fully half the width. With the legs maintaining the six-beat rhythm, perform one complete cycle of arm action, ie *pull, pull, stop*. The arms should commence their pull on the first and fourth beats of the leg rhythm. You can time this into your leg-rhythm count, by accenting the count, thus, 'ONE, *two, three*, FOUR, *five, six*.' Do remember that this does not carry an accentuated leg kick with it.

Doing this exercise, you should feel yourself moving smoothly through the water as the arms pull. A well-swum crawl done at medium speed is sheer poetry in motion to watch. You cannot see yourself, but you should feel yourself doing the action smoothly and easily. When it feels like that, and not until, try extending it. Push off, get the legs going, and when halfway across the width with the legs going well, add two arm-action cycles, ie *pull, pull, pull, pull, stop*. Now increase the number of arm cycles to four, but do bear in mind that it is pointless to carry on practising leg action plus arm action unless the legs are maintaining an efficient action, in the correct rhythm.

Having got this far, let us have a look at this arm action, to make sure that it is being performed correctly. The finger tips should enter the water first. In order to do this, the elbow must be at a higher level than the hand as entry is made. The whole arm should be almost straight, with just sufficient bend to allow the elbow to be lifted higher than the hand. The point of entry should be straight ahead of the shoulder, and certainly no further inward than straight ahead of the nose.

As soon as the hand is in the water you should be feeling for a purchase on the water. Keep the hand as big and flat as you can without spreading the fingers. You will find the purchase on the water at a point about six inches beneath the surface. This is called the 'catch point'. From this point on, the hand should be powered directly backward through the water with the arm straight or nearly so. Remember that at bottom dead centre the action changes from pull to push, and you must go right through with the push until you start to recover the arm. When I speak of powering the hand through the water, this does not presuppose a fast action, but it does mean feeling the hand working against the resistance of the water right through the propulsive phase of the stroke. To do this, the angle of the hand to the forearm must continually vary throughout the propulsive phase in order to keep the hand working directly backward against the water.

Going back to Newton and his laws of motion (*See Chapter 2*), the third law says that to every action there will be an equal and opposite reaction. There are times in swimming when some upward propulsion is deliberately sought – as in the Dolphin Butterfly stroke – but, never, ever, in Crawl. It is in order to maintain the reaction to the arm action in the form of

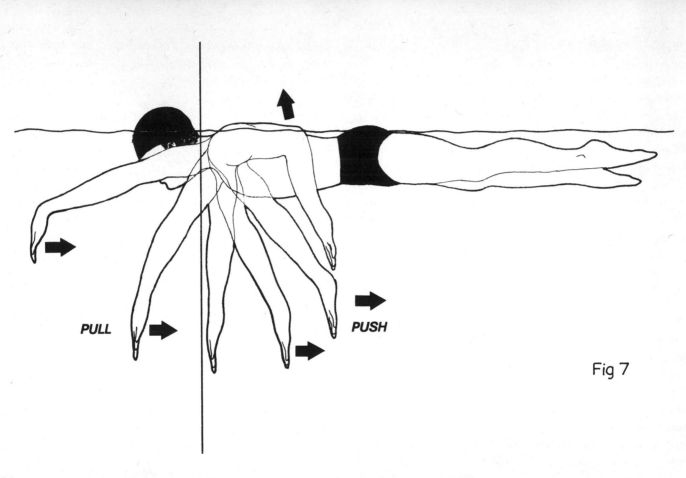

PULL

PUSH

Fig 7

purely forward movement that we try to keep the hand working backward against the water. (*See Fig 7.*)

At the end of the propulsive phase the arm must be lifted clear of the water (with the elbow leading the rest of the arm) and thrown forward to the entry position. Whether this is done as a high 'over the top' action or as a low 'out and round' action is not really important. The important thing is that while the arm is being recovered you have the opportunity to relax the muscles which have worked hard to pull and push it through the propulsive phase. Try to achieve this relaxation by throwing the arm through the recovery as loosely as possible.

By now you should be thinking in terms of a smooth and easy action. Crawl, well performed, is a very beautiful series of movements, and the basis of this beauty is the smooth and flowing quality of the movement. So, before we go on to the breathing technique, you need to get a lot of practice at swimming widths, full stroke, on a held breath. You will be surprised how easily you will achieve a good-looking and effective stroke. This is because you are maintaining a good flat body-position because of an effective leg-action, and not ruining it by lifting your head in an attempt to breathe. Before we go on to breathing, re-read Chapter 2 and remember what happens when you have more than the permitted 1 per cent out of the water. Your head is certainly more than 1 per cent of your body mass!

To summarise the legs-and-arms exercises:

1   Push and glide, add leg action, then add one arm cycle and stop.

2   As for (1), but add two arm cycles and stop.

3   As for (1), but add four arm cycles and stop.

4   As for (1), but add arm action for the remainder of the width.

5   As for (4), concentrating on (a) entry position and posture of hand; (b) the path of the arm through the water; (c) the push, following the pull; (d) varying the angle of hand to forearm in order to maintain backward pressure on the water, and (e) the recovery.

6   Widths, legs and arms, concentrating on a smooth and easy action.

Breathing

It is absolutely essential that you understand the

principles of Crawl breathing, otherwise you could ruin the whole thing and discourage yourself tremendously by deciding that it might be possible to breathe by lifting the head.

Crawl breathing is done via the mouth (explosive technique, preferably), with the mouth at or even fractionally below the normal surface level. Thus it is not necessary to lift the head even a fraction of an inch. The head is merely turned. If, in a standing position, you turn your head until your lower jaw just touches your shoulder, this demonstrates the head action required.

I hope that you are now wondering just how it is possible to inhale air, and not water, from surface level or even below it. Well, what happens is this. When any type of body, human or otherwise, is moved forward on the surface of water, it pushes a pile of water ahead of it. Although we have established that we swim through water, not on it, part of the head will be above the surface, and it is this which pushes the pile of water along. Those who design ships are fortunate in that they can build the vessel with a sharp end which cuts through the water and divides the bow wave, thus minimising resistance. Humans, however, have heads which are rounded and thus cannot cut through the water. So, when we swim, we continually push the pile of water ahead of us. This is why the push and glide is so efficient. The extended arms can divide the water and minimise the resistance.

Although pushing a pile of water along with your head is one of the resistance factors which makes swimming a very mechanically inefficient method of human movement, the great advantage of the situation is that it does allow you to inhale air without lifting your head clear of the surface and ruining the body position. The pile of water had to come from some-where. It wasn't there on the surface before you started to move forward. It has come from where your head has just been, and thus a 'trough' is left in the water on either side of the head. It is from this trough that we get the air to breathe. Of course, the trough fills fairly quickly, thus timing is important. (*See Fig 8*.) It is fortunate that the nature of the arm action is such that it causes a slight rolling of the trunk from side to side. It rolls toward the pulling arm, so that if the head is held in its natural line then the mouth is coming up toward the surface as the arm pulls without any turn at the neck taking place. If, then, at the highest point of the upward roll, the head is turned slightly, the mouth will be clear of the water, the level of which has been

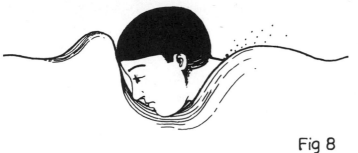

Fig 8

depressed because of the 'trough'.

The point in the arm action where the head is turned and exhalation/inhalation takes place is just before the arm starts its recovery, right at the end of the propulsive action. Turn the head toward the pulling arm, breathe *out-in* and immediately return the head to its natural line.

I hope I have established the point that it is only when forward movement is taking place that it is hydrostatically possible for the conditions to exist in which the correct breathing action can take place. It could not be done in the push and glide position because it is the hands, not the head, which are creating the bow wave, and thus the 'trough' would be filled long before

the head passed through that piece of water. Under these circumstances you would inhale water. Neither can it be done in a stationary position, due to the lack of a bow wave.

Let's do it, then. Take a deep breath, push away from the side and start swimming full stroke. About halfway across the width, turn the head toward the arm that is finishing its propulsive phase and breathe. It does not matter which side you use. With explosive technique, as you blow out you will know whether or not your mouth is sufficiently clear of the water to be able to inhale. If it·is – inhale. If it's not – don't, just centre your head and swim another couple of strokes and then stand up and get some air. You will have to experiment with this quite a bit to get the timing right, but all you are after is one exhale/inhale per width. If it comes right, do not be tempted, yet, to try to breathe once every arm cycle. This has to be built up in the same way that we built up the arm action.

Once you can take your one breath successfully, try taking two per width. The thing is that you do not have to take a breath at any given point, you've already got an adequate supply of air from the deep breath that you took before pushing off. You will probably find that you will still be mistiming it occasionally, but this doesn't matter provided you are using the explosive breathing technique. The forcible exhalation will blow away any water that is around your mouth, and you will not take any in. Actually, it is no bad thing, once you are confident, if a little water does come into your mouth. If it does, let it stay there until the next breath, and then expel it with the air as you forcibly exhale. There was a time, many years ago, when swimming with a mouthful of water for, say, a width, was considered a good training exercise. I wouldn't go all the way with this theory, but it's not a bad confidence exercise.

Now that you are swimming the full stroke, with breathing, do not forget to do a few widths using your legs only from time to time. It's good for your stroke, and good for your figure.

Your first attempts at rhythmic breathing should be by use of alternate breathing. That is, one breath to each two complete stroke-cycles. This is a technique adopted by many competitive swimmers in order to cut down on the number of head movements and thus minimise adverse effects upon body position. For the learner, its advantage is that while you are still at the stage where you are having to think a bit about what you are doing, it gives you a little more time between breathing actions in which to do your thinking. From alternate breathing, move on to breathing every stroke cycle, which is the timing used by most swimmers.

Before leaving the subject of breathing, it should be interesting for you to watch the variations of breathing techniques used by swimmers when you see them in competition. Watch the way that the sprinters usually take only one breath, or even no breath at all, as they swim the first length. They breathe as they turn, and then swim for a considerable distance before breathing again, and eventually adopt a breathing rhythm of one breath to every five or six cycles. Watch also the way that, in a close finish, the contestants do not breathe at all over the last ten yards or so. All this in the interests of preserving body position! Notice the variations of breathing timings used by long-distance swimmers. Some breathe once for every stroke cycle, some use alternate breathing, while some use a technique called 'bilateral breathing', whereby they breathe once every one and a half stroke cycles, so that breath is taken alternately to the left and right. This way, they can keep an eye on opponents on both sides of them.

To summarise exercises for full stroke with breathing:

1 Widths, legs and arms, concentrating on a smooth and easy action, no breathing.

2 One width, attempting to take one breath while swimming, by turning the head, but not lifting it even a fraction of an inch.

3 Build this up to two, three or four breaths per width.

4 Widths, taking one breath every two arm cycles. (Alternate breathing.)

5 Widths, taking one breath each arm cycle.

5 Back Crawl

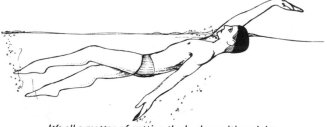

It's all a matter of getting the body position right

Back Crawl should be easy because in doing the Crawl exercises you will have covered practically all the necessary leg work.

Once more, as always, we are looking for a near-horizontal body position, so we start by revising the back push and glide, in the same way as we did when mastering the basics. As you are doing this, hold your head in such a position that you may comfortably watch your feet. This may cause the hips to sink a little, but provided this sinking is not too great it does not matter very much. (*See Fig 9.*)

Leg action

We need the same six-beat rhythms as for Crawl. The legs want to be stretched but not rigid, with the ankles as relaxed as you can get them. You have the great

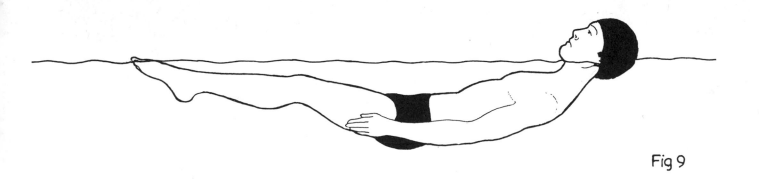

Fig 9

advantage, in Back Crawl, of being able to see your legs while you are practising or swimming full stroke, so there is no excuse for not doing this one well in a short time.

The first practice, then, begins with back push and glide. As soon as you are fully horizontal in the water, start the legs going, and complete the width. Flippers, if permitted, are very useful for this, but do bear in mind that you are going backwards fairly fast and cannot see where you are going.

Ensure, by watching them, that neither your knees nor your feet come out of the water. Your big toes should just break the surface, leaving a turbulence on the water behind them. If your legs are straight, you'll hardly see your knees, and if you do, they will be flat. If you see a rounded knee, push your legs out straight.

Keep your hips well up to the surface. They do have a tendency to sink, and it may be necessary to arch the back very slightly to keep them up.

This exercise may be varied by carrying it out in the following different ways:

With a float under each arm.

With a float held against the lower part of the chest.

With a float held with arms extended beyond the head.

41

With arms by the side.

With arms folded.

With arms by the side, gently sculling with the hands (using the hands as oars).

With the arms extended beyond the head. Do not be depressed if you cannot manage this one – I know some very good swimmers who cannot.

Remember that it is the relaxation of the ankles which promotes propulsion. What you are trying to do, and should work toward feeling yourself doing, is to push against the water with the top surface of the foot as the leg does the upward kick. Remember also that it is the leg action which maintains your body position, and in Back Crawl the arm action wreaks all sorts of havoc in terms of rolling and lateral deviation which only a sound leg action can control.

To summarise the leg action exercises:

1   Revise back push and glide.

2   Back push and glide; when fully horizontal, start legs going.

3   Widths, legs only, using variations of use of floats and arm positions and concentrating on a loose ankle-action.

Arm action

I wish that I could tell you that Back Crawl arm action is just Crawl done upside down, but there is a bit more to it than that. The actions are similar, and have many things in common, but there is one very important difference. Let me explain it by use of the standing position.

If you stand with one arm by your side and the other extended straight upward, and perform the Crawl arm action, the propelling arm moves forward and downward, while the recovering arm moves upward and backward. Both arms are, more or less, moving in the same plane all the time. For Back Crawl, however, from the same standing position, the propelling arm moves outward and downward while the recovering arm moves upward and backward. In fact, one arm is moving in a different plane from the other. Put another way, the propelling arm travels the long way round while the recovering arm goes the shortest way home. (*See Fig 10.*)

This is one of the few instances where an exercise

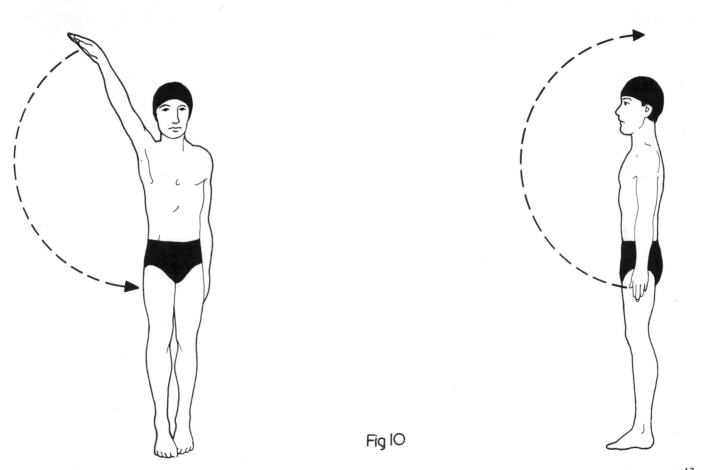

Fig 10

43

done out of the water is very useful. It is worthwhile to spend a few minutes standing in front of a full-length mirror and doing the action, to ensure that you have got the limb track right.

In the water, build up the leg and arm action exercises as we did for Crawl. First, push off, get the legs going and, when you are halfway across the width, do one complete arm cycle and stop. Remember that the arms enter on the first and fourth beats of the leg rhythm. Build this up to two arm-cycles, then three, then four, bearing in mind as you do so that this, like Crawl, is a continuous arm action; as the propelling arm completes its action, it must be whipped very smartly out of the water and into the recovery. You may have worked out by now that the propulsion phase is going to take longer than the recovery. It is necessary for the pro-pelling arm to be well into the water by the time the other arm comes out, in order to keep the arms in 180 degree opposition.

At this point, let us have a look at the arm action with a view to getting it right. Ideally the hand should enter, with the little finger leading and with the arm fully extended, at a point immediately behind the shoulder. Both arms in this position would give you a 'five minutes to one' situation, using a clock-face analogy. Do not strain to reach this position, however, if you cannot achieve it comfortably. The entry may be efficiently done further out, but not beyond the 'ten minutes to two' position. Start feeling for a purchase on the water as soon as the hand is in, dropping the hand on the wrist in order to do so. Having made the entry and found a 'catch', the procedure may seem a lot more complicated than it really is, but if you follow the description with reference to Fig 11 it should be quite clear:

The arm is pulled around from the catch point to a point opposite the shoulder.

From the point opposite the shoulder, the arm is allowed to sink down until the hand is opposite the hip. Thus the plane of the action has altered slightly.

As the hand travels beyond the hip, the arm is now sweeping upward toward the surface. Just before the hand reaches the surface, the palm is turned outward, in order that the hand may leave the water with the little finger leading.

As in Crawl, the angle of the hand on the wrist should

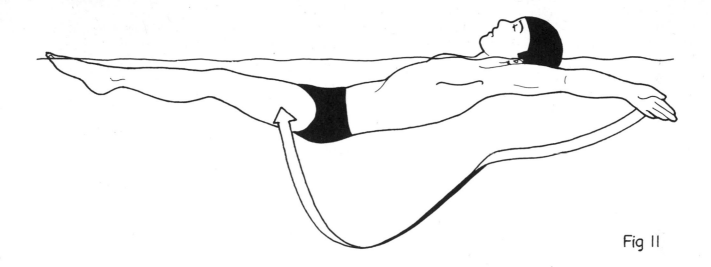

Fig 11

vary as the arm travels through its arc, in order to maintain directly forward pressure against the water, thus obtaining maximum backward propulstion.

To summarise the leg-action and arm-action exercises:

1   Widths, legs only, with arms by the sides.

2   Widths, legs only, adding one cycle of arm action per width. Concentrate on making the arm action continuous, which necessitates a fast transition from the end of the propulsive phase to the recovery phase.

3   Widths, adding two, three and four arm-actions, concentrating on (a) entry at the 'five minutes to one' position, little finger first; (b) pull round, push down,

up and out; (c) turning the hand to a palm-outward position at the end of the 'push' element of the propulsive phase, so that the little finger can leave the water first; and (d) varying the angle of the hand to the forearm in order to maintain a directly backward pressure against the water.

4   Widths, full stroke, working for a smooth and easy action.

Fortunately there are no breathing problems in Back Crawl. The face is clear of the water throughout. The only possible problem might be that of water dripping on to the face as the recovering arm comes over, but if you use the explosive breathing technique you will blow away any water that is near your lips before inhaling.

Now you can start to build up to a full-stroke swimming situation by swimming widths. Push off, get the legs going and, as soon as they are working well, bring the arms in and complete the width. The great thing is that in Back Crawl full stroke should feel really smooth. If it does not feel smooth and easy, it is probable either that you have allowed your hips to drop or that your legs are not working efficiently.

As with Crawl, do not neglect to keep your leg practices going just because you've started swimming full stroke. As in all strokes, the arm action becomes very difficult if your body position is not right. It is the leg action which keeps you in the near-horizontal position, and you have to work at it.

6   Breast Stroke

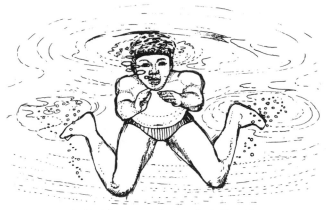

I didn't know you had to do it like this

This chapter would perhaps be more aptly called 'Breast Strokes', since there are two permissible versions of the stroke – not counting the Dolphin Butterfly stroke. These are variously known as 'old style' and 'new style', 'head up' and 'head down', 'diamond kick' and 'W-kick' etc. Some competitive swimmers use a mixture of both styles, so it's a reasonably open game for the learner. The thing to bear in mind, however, is that if one wishes to acquire a good Breast Stroke, and it is generally the best stroke to use if one wants to swim for any significant distance, then the optimum mechanical efficiency will be obtained by doing it in the prescribed manner. I use the word 'prescribed' quite deliberately, since the laws of swimming lay down quite specific requirements for the stroke. Briefly, the body must be kept perfectly on the breast, with both

47

shoulders in line with the surface, and movements of either arms or legs must be simultaneous and symmetrical.

It has always seemed to me that if people learn to swim the stroke according to the laws, which are nothing more than a description of the classically correct method of swimming the stroke, they can then modify their techniques to suit their individual differences when they become proficient. So we will start with the traditional version of the stroke, and go on to the modern modifications.

The body position is, as always, as near to the horizontal as we can get it, although the legs are lower in the water than is normal in push and glide. Arm and leg actions will alter the body position considerably throughout the stroke cycle, but we will be trying all the time to maintain this near-horizontal position. Revise the push and glide exercises to perfect the basic position. Repeat the push and glide with the head held so that the surface of the water is at approximately eyebrow level instead of across the top of the head. This means raising the head very, very slightly, which in turn will cause the legs to sink equally slightly, giving the body position a slight slope from the shoulders down to the feet.

Leg action

Starting from the push and glide position, where the legs are together and extended, the heels should be drawn up, the knees pushing as they bend, until they reach the seat. Thus, the legs are in the form of a diamond (*See Fig 12*) with the feet in a 'flat foot' position and turned as far outward as they will go.

From the 'diamond' position the feet are pushed outward and backward until the legs are almost straight, at which point the legs are brought together and back to the push and glide position. As the legs are brought together, the feet resume their stretched and pointed position. The propulsion is gained by the reaction to the powerful backward pressure of the soles of the feet against the water. Since the bulk of Breast Stroke propulsion comes from the leg action, it is necessary to perfect this action, and particularly to get the feel of the soles of the feet pushing back against the water.

The first exercise should be carried out while lying horizontally in the water, grasping the rail. Move the legs slowly through the pattern described, to a count of *2, 3*. Draw the legs up on *2*, and sweep them out and round on *3*. The count of *2, 3* is useful in that it gives a good (but not perfect) indication of the timing of the full stroke, when we get there.

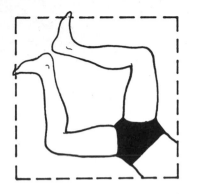

Fig 12

Next, push and glide, preferably holding a float. When you have achieved the near-horizontal position, remembering that the water should be at eyebrow level, start the legs going to a count of *2, 3, 4*. As you did at the rail, recover the legs on *2*, kick round and back on *3*, and hold the push and glide position on *4*.

As you progress with this exercise, you must try to make the recovery and the kick of legs into a continuous movement, with no pause at all between the two elements. Thus, the rhythm will become *2, 3 – 4*, with *2* running into *3*, but with a slight pause before *4*, which should not be difficult, since on *4* you do nothing but glide through the water.

Once you get the feel of the glide resulting from the powerful leg action, it is better to do the practice without a float. Just push and glide, and pick up the leg action as soon as you are gliding. Continue this for as long as your breath holds out. You should also practise this on the back, starting with back push and glide. In this position you are able to see your legs, and can check visually that your action is correct. This is also a good practice in its own right, since it will be useful for Backstroke later.

Try to push and glide underwater, and complete the width using your legs only. Keep your arms extended ahead of you to save your head, should you collide with anything or anybody.

Do the same practice from push and glide, but this time with a float held vertically to provide some resistance against which to strengthen your leg action. It will cut your glide down very considerably, but it will make you work harder with your legs, which is all to the good.

The really important things to think about while doing these exercises are:

Force the thighs outward to get the knees as wide apart as possible. It is important that both knees are lifted to the same degree, so that the position is symmetrical, and not skewed.

Turning the feet outward as far as they will go, immediately before starting the kick.

Keep working away at these exercises until your leg kick is really efficient. Given a good push and glide to begin with you should, by really holding the glide after each leg kick, manage a width of the average swimming pool in two or three leg actions.

Get someone to watch you, to ensure that your leg action is entirely symmetrical and, if it is not, to tell you which knee must be lifted to achieve symmetry. This business of the 'screwkick' is quite prevalent (*See Fig 13*), and for every swimmer who does it because he is not aware that his legs are not forming a symmetrical pattern, and who can thus cure it by lifting one knee more, there are six swimmers who get one knee higher than the other in the diamond position

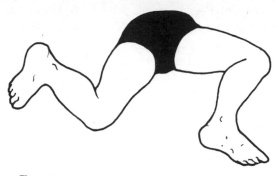

Fig 13

because they have one hip joint which is more supple than the other. In the latter case, any attempt to raise the offending knee higher will cause the whole hip girdle to turn, thus rendering a symmetrical kick impossible. Such people should try to achieve symmetry by lowering the 'good' knee to the level of the 'bad' one, rather than vice versa.

Arm action

Most people who can swim Breast Stroke 'a bit' sweep the arms around far too widely. Breast Stroke

50

has a fairly short arm-action, which also goes rather deeper than most people appreciate. From the extended position of the push and glide, the arms are pulled downward and backward over a distance of about twenty inches – and no more. A good rough-and-ready guide for this is that if your head is still, with the eyes looking straight ahead, you can see your hands in the starting position. Keeping the eyes looking straight ahead, pull downward and backward until they disappear from your sight. When they disappear, you have gone too far. The entire arm action is carried out with the hands visible while looking straight ahead. This is movement *1*, the propulsive phase.

Recovery of the arms begins at the end of the propulsive phase. The arms are pulled inward, elbows leading, until the upper arms are against the chest with the hands pointing forward. This is movement *2*, the first part of the recovery. From here, the arms are pushed straight forward to the push and glide position. This is movement *3*, the second part of the recovery. The final phase of the arm action is merely to rest in the push and glide position. This is movement *4*, and in this position you glide through the water taking every advantage of the powerful leg action which, you will remember, came at movement *3*. Thus, the rhythm of the arm action is *1-2, 3-4*. *2* and *3* merge together into one continuous recovery movement.

To fit leg and arm actions together, start from push and glide. Get the legs going and, when halfway across the width, add two arm cycles to the leg actions, and then stop. It is probable that the first arm action will not synchronise too well with the leg action, but the second should go well. Build this up to three arm actions, then four, until you can go easily and smoothly across the width.

Breathing

On movement *1* of the arm action, the arms pull downward and backward. According to Newton's third law, the reaction to this action will be upward and forward (equal and opposite). The forward reaction is good, since it sends the body in the direction in which we want it to go. In this case, the upward reaction is also good, in that it will propel the body upward sufficiently to get the mouth clear of the water with only a minimal raising of the head. At the end of the first part of the arm movement, then, the water will be at or about chin level. It is at this point, at the end of the propulsive action of the arms, that breathing takes place. The explosive technique is recommended, because the held breath will help to minimise the sinking which is bound to follow the lifting of the head out of the water. For this type of stroke, which incorporates a long gliding action, one breath per stroke cycle is usual. As soon as the breathing action is completed, the head should be returned to its previous position, with the water surface at about the level of the eyebrows.

The new-style Breast Stroke

This is widely used among competitive swimmers, and the main points of deviation from the older, classical gliding style are as follows:

The head is held high – clear of the water at all times. There is thus no lifting and lowering of the head in order to breathe, which keeps the body position much more stable by avoiding the undulation of the whole body which invariably accompanies head movement.

The legs are recovered into a 'W' shape, rather than a diamond, and are never brought together at the end of the leg action.

The arm action is shorter and shallower. Since the upper body does not need to be lifted to enable breathing

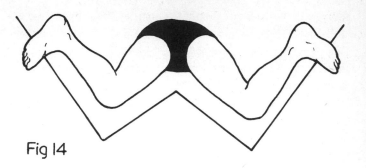

Fig 14

to take place, there is no need for a downward element in the arm action.

There is no glide; leg action is continuous.

If you would like to try this style of Breast Stroke swimming, the points of technique that you will need to practise are given below.

Leg Action

From the push and glide position, the legs are drawn up with the knees apart, but held quite low – about 90 degrees to the trunk, but with the feet wide of the hips, in the flat foot position. From the rear, the legs form a 'W' shape. (*See Fig 14.*) The feet and legs are driven straight back, with the inside of the foot and of the lower leg pushing back against the water. As the legs straighten, they are immediately recovered and kicked again. The rhythm is a simple *bend, kick, bend, kick, bend, kick*. For those who have no wish to do a fast breast stroke, this pattern of leg movement is very easy, especially for those who are unable to achieve symmetry in the diamond position, and it can be used within the *1-2, 3-4* rhythm of traditional Breast Stroke.

Arm action

This is almost a continuous circling movement. After the pull, the entire recovery movement is aimed only at getting the arms back to the extended position as quickly as possible, in order to start another pull. Remember, too, that the legs are working on a simple two-beat rhythm, so the arms have got to do likewise in order to co-ordinate the stroke as a whole.

Thus movement *1* is as before, except that there is almost no downward element in the movement – it is almost purely backward, and it is shorter – only about 12–15 inches from start to finish. At the end of the pull, movement *2* is nothing but an inward rotation of the hands to turn the palms downward as the arms are pushed forward. The timing is a simple *1, 2, 1, 2, 1, 2*. As the arms pull, the legs recover, on *1*. The arms recover as the legs kick, on *2*. Remember that the head is held clear of the water throughout, so no head movement is necessary when breathing.

If you intend to try this, try it in short bursts – widths rather than lengths. It is a bit energetic, and, until you have got the co-ordination right, will be really hard work.

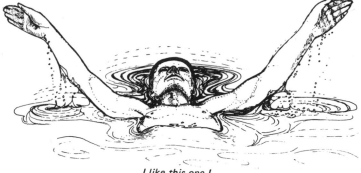

I like this one !

7   Backstroke

English Backstroke, as it is sometimes called, is a most useful stroke to add to your repertoire. One can cover long distances using this stroke without massive calls upon energy. It is unique in that, unlike any other recognised stroke, it has a massively propulsive action from both arms and legs. It is swum on the back with Back Crawl arm-action performed by both arms simultaneously, followed by an inverted Breast Stroke leg-action. The body position is as near to the horizontal as possible, with the head carried on the natural line, although some prefer to hold the head forward a little.

Leg action

This is exactly as for Breast Stroke, except that it may be necessary not to draw the legs up too far, in order to prevent the knees from coming out of the water. Swim widths, legs only, from the back push and glide position, concentrating on getting the feel of really pushing against the water with the inside of the foot and calf. The rhythm for the leg action is *bend, kick, glide; bend, kick, glide*. This should be done with the arms at the sides.

Arm action

From the back push and glide position, both arms are thrown up and back to enter the water, little finger leading, at a 'five minutes to one' position, using the analogy of a clock face. As soon as entry is made, feel for a purchase on the water; having obtained it, pull the arms round until the palms meet the thighs.

The only difficulty in fitting this arm action to the leg action lies in the timing, since this is a two-phase stroke, where each glide from both the arm and leg action is separately used.

Swim with your legs only, and add the arm action when halfway across the width, using the following rhythm: (legs) *bend, kick, glide*, (arms) *throw, pull, glide*. What we have is a six-beat rhythm, composed of recovery, propulsion and glide for both arms and legs.

Since the face is clear of the water, there are no breathing difficulties.

People do this for pleasure ?

8 Butterfly

For most swimmers the Butterfly stroke has a sort of gruesome fascination. In order to swim Butterfly with sufficient ease to cover any appreciable distance, the swimmer needs physical characteristics which most adults no longer possess, or perhaps never possessed. The first is a high degree of suppleness in the shoulder joints. You can test your own shoulder mobility by standing with your arms hanging by your sides and circling both arms together, first by circling them from front to back to loosen up (*Fig 15*) and then the real test, from back to front (*Fig 16*).

The further backward and upward you can swing your arms while still keeping them parallel with each other, the more supple are your shoulder joints. Most of us find that in order to make a circle it is necessary to start moving the arms outward almost as soon as

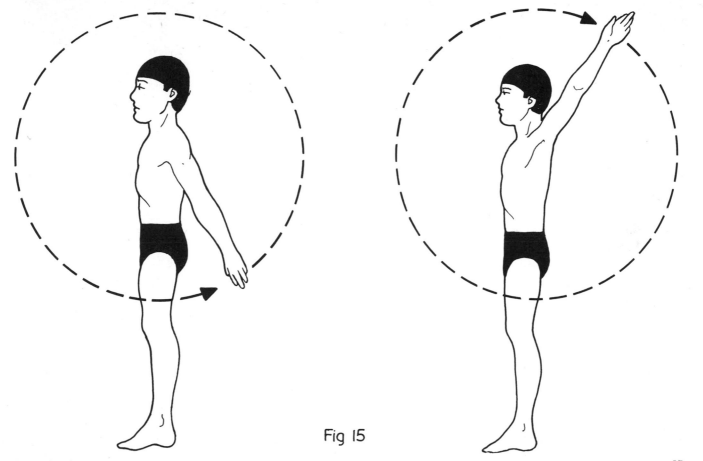

Fig 15

we start the upswing. To swim this stroke well, and with relative ease, it is necessary to have the ability to swing the arms upward sufficiently far to get them clear of the water before allowing them to move outward.

If you are one of the vast majority who lack this high degree of suppleness, this need not prevent you from having a little fun trying the stroke. You may do a width, and probably a length, if you don't mind puffing and grunting a bit, but it is doubtful whether you'll ever be invited to join the national training squad. It is, however, a source of great personal satisfaction to be able to perform, even if only over a short distance, a stroke which most people consider to be the exclusive preserve of the expert swimmer.

In essence, the stroke has a co-ordination which is made up of two complete leg actions (while the arms are pulling through the water) followed by the over-the-water recovery of the arms, which, for practical purposes gives a stroke rhythm of *beat, beat, throw; beat, beat, throw; beat, beat, throw* and so on, and it is vital to get the *beat, beat*, of the legs right before trying to add an arm action.

Body position

As in all strokes, the ideal is to keep as near to the

horizontal as possible, but in Butterfly the combination of the leg and arm actions causes the body to undulate like a dolphin, which is why the stroke used to be called the Dolphin Butterfly. However, you do start in a near-horizontal position and, given any luck at all, return to it at the end of every stroke cycle. The main thing for the learner to know is that, like Crawl, it is swum with the head held on its natural line, which means face in the water, except for that part of the stroke cycle when, as in Breast Stroke, the reaction to limb actions lifts the head clear of the water and breathing takes place.

Leg action

This is very much like the Crawl leg action performed with both legs simultaneously, the main difference being that there is a slight bending of the knees as the legs move up and down. If it is permitted, do try to wear a pair of flippers while doing the exercises. They make it all much easier, and make it possible for you to get the 'feel' of the stroke quite quickly. Once you have this 'feel', you will be able to go quite well without the flippers.

1   Take a deep breath. Push and glide. As soon as you are horizontal in the water, start the legs going, saying to yourself 'Beat, beat, pause; beat, beat, pause'.

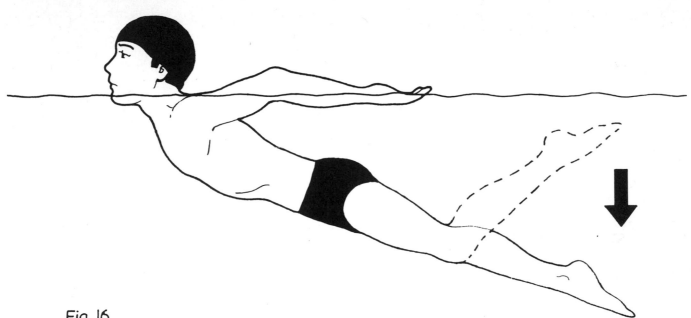

Fig 16

2 Repeat (1), emphasising the first of the two leg beats – ie *BEAT*, *beat*, *pause*. In the full stroke the first leg action is the major beat – the really powerful one which drives you forward through the water – while the second is the minor beat which lifts the head and shoulders, enabling the arms to be lifted out of the water in order that they may be thrown forward. (*See Fig 16*.)

3 Take a deep breath. Push and glide to the bottom of the pool and repeat (2) underwater. Keep your arms extended ahead of you – and keep your eyes open. If the leg action has become efficient, and you are wearing flippers, you move at a fair speed when underwater, and if you collide with someone's legs, or ram into the wall, it's not very pleasant!

Do not bother with breathing techniques yet. Do each width, or as much of it as you can manage, on a held breath. You may notice when watching Butterfly swimmers that the hips move up and down as they kick, giving a marked undulating effect to the lower trunk. Do not try to copy this while practising leg action, since this undulation is not a deliberately acquired movement. It is the reaction of the hips to those phases of the stroke when both arms and legs are moving up or down at the same time, in the same way that bending both ends of a ruler upward and downward would produce the opposite reaction in the middle.

Arm action

Since we are only trying the Butterfly for fun, there is little point in flogging away at leg exercises until the action is nearly perfect in the same way that I've suggested for the other strokes. Once you can get across two or three widths using your legs only, have a go at the full stroke. The arm action is very much like that of Crawl, except that both arms work together, symmetrically and simultaneously.

The hands enter the water fingers first and about shoulder width apart, or perhaps a little wider, according to how supple the shoulders are. As the hands enter, the arms should be bent slightly, so that at the moment of entry the elbows are held higher than the hands. (*See Fig 17*.) As soon as the hands are in the water, pull downward and backward and inward until the arms are pointing directly downward (towards the bottom of the pool). At this point, change the pulling action to a pushing action and push the arms backward and outward. Thus, the arms are following a 'tailor's dummy', or 'hourglass' path. The arms will bend as

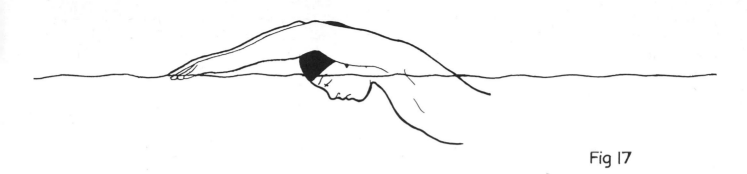

Fig 17

they are powered through the water, and at the end of the push phase the palms should be turned inward to allow the hands to come out of the water smoothly and with streamlining. As soon as they are clear of the water, the arms are thrown over to the entry position. The higher you can lift them in the recovery, the better; but this, again, depends on your shoulder mobility. It also requires a fair amount of shoulder strength to be able to keep this continuous arm circling going at a speed fast enough to achieve the correct stroke rhythm of *beat, beat, THROW; beat, beat, THROW*. You will probably find that you have to allow a little pause for a glide before you begin the next pull, which doesn't matter unless you want to achieve a perfect stroke.

Let's try the whole thing, then. Push off and glide. Start the legs going – *beat, beat, pause*. As soon as the legs are going well, add the arm action, starting the first pull on the first of the two leg-beats, which will bring your arms through to the start of the recovery movement immediately after the second leg-beat, giving a rhythm of *beat, beat, THROW*.

If you find the going a bit too hard initially, and the whole thing does not fit together nicely, try doing it with this rhythm: *beat, beat, THROW; beat, beat, pause; beat, beat, THROW; beat, beat, pause*. By doing this, you will be doing the arm action once in every two stroke-cycles, instead of doing it every stroke-cycle, and the alternate glide in the push-and-glide position will give you time to recover a good body position in which to do the next arm action. If you practise this for a while you should soon work up to the correct full stroke, but don't worry if you never do the full stroke, it's a stroke that not everyone is able to do, and we only decided to try it for a bit of fun in the first place.

To sum up, the Butterfly exercises are:

1   Push and glide, with leg action, to a rhythm of 'beat, beat, pause'.

2   Repeat, emphasising the first of the two leg-beats but using the same basic rhythm.

3   Repeat (2) underwater.

4   Plenty of widths of (2). Wear flippers if you are able.

5   Push and glide, get legs going, and add arm action, using the rhythm *beat*, *beat*, *THROW*.

6   If (5) proves too demanding, use the arm action only on alternate stroke-cycles.

7   Full stroke practice over short distances.

Hopefully, you will have no breathing problems once you start on full stroke. You will find that the second leg-beat tends to lift your face and shoulders clear of the water, and you can take a breath as your arms are coming out of the water at the beginning of the recovery phase. In case your co-ordination of the stroke isn't as good as it might be, always take a good lungful of air before you start, so that you do not get desperate and have to stop for breath just when things are going together nicely. Avoid, if you possibly can, throwing your head up in order to breathe. If you do so, the action of lifting the head quickly initiates a 'porpoising' action which, in addition to making the stroke much more difficult, affords considerable amusement to any of your friends who happen to be watching.

Don't be put off by all this technical stuff – have a go. Only a fool would try to pretend that Butterfly is an easy stroke to swim, but it is fun trying, and it is most satisfying to be able to produce a reasonable facsimile of the stroke, even if only for a width.

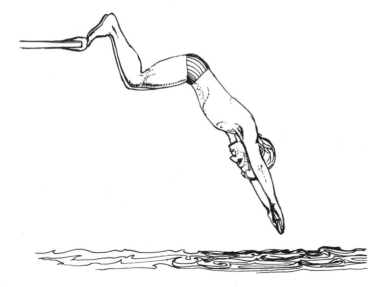

9 Diving

Anyone who is taking the trouble to try to improve his swimming owes it to himself to learn to dive neatly, if not spectacularly. The plunge dive most of us can manage, since it is little more than falling into the water head first, and one of the objects of the plunge dive is to meet the water as far away from the take off as possible. Thus the racing start is only a sophistication of the humble plunge dive.

If, however, you wish to dive from either fixed boards or spring-boards, no matter how low, a rather different technique is necessary. Fortunately, diving technique is fairly easy to learn. If you are nervous about diving, start by standing in the pool, in water slightly more than waist deep.

Stance

Stand on the pool side, at a place where the water is

about eighteen inches deeper than your own height. Stand with your feet together, toes curled over the edge, with big toes, ankles and knees together. Your legs should be straight, your trunk upright, and your eyes looking straight ahead. Extend your arms above your head, with your hands about two feet apart. You are now in the 'Y' position, from which all dives start.

Take off

At take off, you are attempting to project yourself upward, not outward. If your take off is correct, you will enter the water no more than eighteen inches ahead of your take off. This is the important difference between plunging and diving. Watch people at the pool using the boards. The vast majority fall forward, and it is not until the whole body is nearly horizontal that the feet lose contact with the board. They generally meet the water six to eight feet from the board. It's fun, which justifies it entirely, but it is not diving.

The take off should be an upward motion. In order to get a good take off and avoid clobbering yourself on the pool side as you go in, try some feet-first entries. Take up the stance (above) and bend the knees and push the bottom backward slightly, without bending the trunk forward. This backward displacement of the

hips will ensure that you travel far enough forward to enter safely. If, however, the body is bent forward from the hips, the direction of travel will be predominantly forward, which is what we are seeking to avoid.

From here, spring upward as vigorously as you can, bringing the arms together and locking the thumbs together, as for push and glide. The object now is to make the body as long, thin and rigid as possible. Everything, neck, trunk, legs, arms, hands and feet should be stretched as hard as possible. In order to achieve a comfortable entry in the feet-first position, fix the eyes on a point on the pool wall opposite, and keep watching it with the head still until the head disappears beneath the water. This precludes pitching forward and slapping the face on the water, which is not terribly harmful but not all that pleasant either.

Entry

This is a matter of putting the extended body through the hole in the water which was made by the first part of the body to meet it – in this case, the feet. Obviously, in order to do this, the body must be near vertical at the moment of entry. This is reasonably easy to achieve from a feet-first entry, provided the body is held rigidly and the head is kept still on its natural line with the body. At the moment of entry the whole body should be rigidly extended with the toes pointed, and this position should be held until the finger tips are submerged.

Practise feet-first entries, working at getting a higher lift at take off, until you are able to enter vertically and fully stretched each and every time. Next, we move to the plain header, which is the dive on which all the others are based.

Take the same stance as before. Push the hips slightly further back on take off, and lift your legs upward and backward quickly as soon as your feet lose contact with the pool side, in order to straighten the body. You should imagine that you are trying to dive over a waist-high fence immediately in front of you.

In flight, keep your upper arms pressing tightly against your ears. Resist the temptation to lift the head. If you do lift your head from between your arms, your hands will make one hole in the water, and your face will make another – which is not very nice. Only by keeping the head between the arms will it pass through the hole already made in the water by the hands. The object is to cause the body to go up, to rotate about the hips until it is upside down, and to drop vertically into the water. Although one should learn and practise this action from the pool side, because from such a low level the impact against the water is minimal should you get it all wrong and land in the belly-flop position, this dive is a lot easier to perform from a raised diving-board, even if only at one metre. The longer flight gives you much more time to rotate the body through the necessary 180 degrees. Before committing yourself to a header from a board, however, no matter how successful your pool side practices have been, try a few feet-first entries. This will give you the feel of the longer drop to the water. Do not, however, attempt to dive from boards into a depth of less than eight feet. An adult, fully extended with arms raised, tends to be anything from seven to eight feet long and, in order to get the full braking effect from the water, the whole body needs to be submerged before the hands come in contact with the bottom of the pool. There are still swimming pools with a maximum depth of six feet or thereabouts that have a diving board or boards, and it is pretty cold comfort when nursing a broken wrist or nose to be able to say that the owners ought to know better!

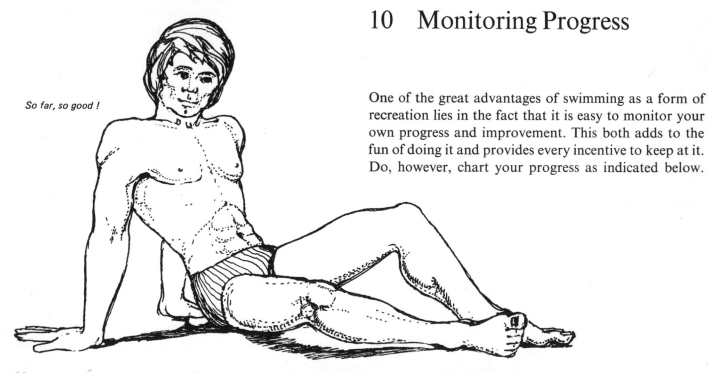

So far, so good !

10   Monitoring Progress

One of the great advantages of swimming as a form of recreation lies in the fact that it is easy to monitor your own progress and improvement. This both adds to the fun of doing it and provides every incentive to keep at it. Do, however, chart your progress as indicated below.

You will be very much more impressed by your improvement in a few months, if it is logged in a form which shows the picture over a period of time.

Note your maximum performance, every two weeks:
Date

Swimming progress

Distance on worst stroke
Distance on second stroke
Distance on best stroke
(Distance should be expressed in lengths or widths, eg 2L=two lengths, 3W=three widths.)

Fitness

Initial measurements   Periodic measurements
Pulse rates per minute
Resting
After maximum swim
After ease down
Normal chest measurement
Waist measurement
Weight

Performance

You should first establish your maximum performance on each stroke, in terms of distance – even if this is as little as a width, or half a width – taking your worst stroke first. This might read:

Back Crawl – *nil* (*can't do it yet*)
Crawl – *1 width*   =*1 width*+*1 length*
Breast Stroke – *1 length*

The three strokes should be swum one after another over the full distance with no break between – the idea being that you swim your worst stroke until you just cannot manage another yard, when you change to your next stroke, and then to your best. It may be that you are so shattered after swimming your worst stroke that you are unable to go on to your next, or your best. In such a case, you should adjust the distance swum on your worst stroke to a point where you have enough energy left to go on to your next stroke and then your best stroke – but you should finish the whole thing feeling thoroughly tired, and unwilling or unable to attempt to go any further. This, then, is your maximum performance, and the measurement you are concerned with is nothing more sophisticated than how shattered you feel at the end of it.

This maximum performance test should be done at the end of every session in the water. I would suggest that at each session you should apportion your time as follows:

5 minutes warm-up.

10–15 minutes stroke training.

5 minutes (maximum) on monitoring progress.

5 minutes ease-down.

The effects of this are usually quite interesting. The first couple of times the maximum performance swim is attempted, the reaction of the average adult would-be improver is – 'Good Heavens! Whatever am I doing this to myself for?' Swimming, done well, is still one of the least mechanically efficient forms of locomotion known to man. Done badly, it requires an awful lot of effort to cover even a short distance, thus the demands in terms of heart work, breathing and power output from muscles are quite considerable and make for pretty heavy exercise, which is, fortunately, done in the ideal position. (*See Chapter I.*) This gives the tyro a vested interest in discovering and utilising the swimming procedures which are least profligate with his energy. He learns that instead of thrashing his way across a width, a good push and glide will get him halfway across with almost no energy expenditure. He learns to let the water support him, instead of fighting it. He thus does two things. He starts to become a better swimmer; he also finds that his maximum performance progressively becomes a task he can manage quite comfortably, and is, in fact, no longer a maximum performance. After a week or ten days he finds that a swim which felt as if it was half killing him can now be done with a considerably reduced energy output, and he realises, with much pleasure, that he is getting better.

Once it has become obvious that the maximum performance is no longer a true maximum, it must be increased to a point where it is again a taxing business, in terms of energy. The increase in performance should be spread across the whole thing, ie an equal increase on all three strokes, say 50 per cent on each. This increased maximum will, again, become progressively easier to do as your bodily systems become more able to meet the demands made upon them and as your strokes become more efficient. Once it becomes easier, increase it again, and carry on doing so until you reach a point where the maximum performance swim is being carried out in lengths, even if your worst stroke is only being swum for one length.

When the maximum swim is being done in lengths, you should then adopt a 'schedule swim', thus:

One length of worst stroke.

Two lengths of best stroke.   = 150 metres

Two lengths of second stroke.

One length of best stroke.

You should adjust this, gradually, until you can swim two lengths using each stroke, one following the other without a break; and when you can do that, you don't need me any more! By the way, when I talk of lengths, I am thinking in terms of a 20–25 metre length. If you are working in a longer pool, adjust the number of lengths accordingly.

If you should want to go on monitoring your performance, the next thing to do is to undertake a five-minute time distance swim. Using each stroke in turn, for one length, establish how many lengths you are able to cover in five minutes. This would include half and quarter lengths. Swim this distance on every visit to the pool until you have done it ten times, and then see if you can push the distance up by half a length, but still within the five-minute period. If you get to this stage, you might well be interested in going for one of the awards mentioned in Appendix B.

Fitness

To monitor the physical benefits that will accrue from your swimming programme, it is necessary to record some information before you start on it. Record the following information as in the table on page 67:

Resting pulse rate. This should be taken when you have been sitting down for half an hour or more, and should be checked on three or four successive days to ensure that you get a normal reading. It should be around seventy-eight per minute.

Chest measurement.

Waist measurement.

Weight is not a very significant factor in the early stages. You will no doubt get rid of some fat, if you are carrying any, but in terms of overall bodyweight this will probably be compensated for by an increase in muscular development, especially about the chest and shoulders. Similarly, the amount your waist measurement decreases will depend to a large extent upon the proportion of your swimming programme which is taken up with swimming on the back. This is a much stronger abdominal exercise than are the strokes swum on the front.

In addition to the above you will need to establish, while at the pool, your pulse rate immediately you finish your maximum-performance swim, and your pulse rate on leaving the water after your ease-down. The pulse rate required to do your maximum swim will decrease as you get used to doing it regularly. Once you increase your maximum, of course, the pulse rate will probably increase as well, but you will observe a steady overall decrease in pulse rate over a period. Your pulse rate should also return to normal more quickly after finishing the maximum-performance swim. Your ease-down activity should take five minutes, which is in effect the first five minutes of your recovery (from exercise) time. The greater the drop in pulse rate over this five minute period, the better.

It should be appreciated that this is only a rule-of-thumb measurement, and that all sorts of other factors affect pulse rate. (The amount you smoke, how long ago you had your last cigarette, your mental and emotional state, etc.) It should, however, provide a good indication of how you are reacting physically. There are other factors which are not easy to measure in this situation. Breathing is one. You will no doubt feel your breathing becoming more efficient. This will be due partly to more efficient swimming techniques which make less demands on breathing, partly to the fact that you are becoming better at the actual business of getting air into you while swimming, but partly due to the fact that your respiratory muscles and your lungs are getting better at their job.

Fitness monitoring should be done fortnightly for the first three months, and monthly thereafter.

11 Teaching a Child to Swim

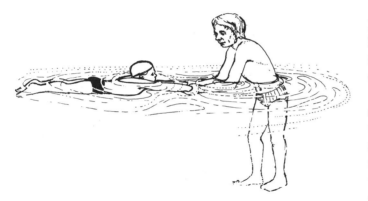

If, as a result of what we have been doing so far, you have met with some success, it is possible that you will think about teaching your own, or someone else's, children to swim.

Whoever first starts teaching a child to swim should try to acquire enough knowledge to ensure that the child is taught well. There is no great mystique about this, although there are those who would attempt to wrap an esoteric cloak around it. It cannot be all that mysterious, since every year hundreds of people – schoolteachers, swimming club helpers, swimming pool attendants, parents, youth club helpers etc – take a course consisting of twelve two-hour sessions, take an examination, and emerge with the Amateur Swimming Association's Teachers' Certificate for Swimming – which is the officially recognised qualification to teach.

With this certificate, many education authorities will employ people as swimming instructors. Many of these people are themselves swimmers of only moderate attainment, since personal performance is not important in teaching swimming, and thus is not included in the syllabus for the examination, except that all are required to demonstrate their ability to effect a simple rescue, and to apply resuscitation procedure.

If, therefore, you are minded to teach a child to swim, do bear in mind the following points. Having done so, you will have done a great service to the child, because unless a parent or friend takes the child on, there is very little possibility that he will ever get individual tuition elsewhere. By far the best pupil/teacher ratio is one to one, and the average child will learn much more quickly in this situation.

When to start

We established very early on in this book that the real essence of good swimming is complete water confidence. This being so, the child really cannot be started too early, provided that all concerned realise that the object of the exercise is simply to give the child water confidence. Mother and baby classes are a marvellous innovation insofar as the young child, surrounded by the security of his mother's arms, in a warm and pleasant environment, is led to discover the joy and pleasure of just being in water. Given the right flotation aids – inflatable armbands are best – the young child can be encouraged to propel himself through the water – again a source of great pleasure to both the parent and the child – but all this is, or should be, no more than one of the earliest confidence practices. It is when well meaning people mistake the willingness and ability of the child to wriggle his way through the water while wearing a pair of armbands for readiness for formalised swimming teaching, that the problems begin. The distribution of the body weight of the very young child renders it impossible for him to achieve a horizontal position. This, in itself, is no great drawback, provided the child's swimming is thought of simply as an exercise in drownproofing and a further step toward water confidence. It is when the child is asked to swim increasing distances in this way, in the belief that this will start him on the road to being a good swimmer, that whoever is teaching him has ceased to do him any favours. Mother and baby classes should be about enjoyment, not about achievement, and you would be wise to give a wide berth to any such group which makes a point of telling you how many one-year-olds can swim the length of the pool, or about how they have a three-year-old who can do ten lengths. Only when the child is confident enough, tall enough (relative to the depth of the water), strong enough, and has a sufficient level of understanding to start on push and glide practices, is it possible to start formally to teach him stroke technique.

Regardless of the age at which a child starts, once he is out of the mother and baby age-bracket, all your efforts should be directed towards getting him to assume the horizontal position in the water, with the face submerged. With the average child you are not going to reach this stage for some time; probably in no less than ten sessions, and often longer than that. The confidence exercises that you should use with a child are much less sophisticated than those suggested for adults in Chapter 2. This has to be so because of the fact that one cannot expect a child to rationalise about the situation in the same way as an adult. The exercises need to be play-based – things which are fun to do.

Confidence exercises

The first test of a child's confidence is whether or not he is willing to get into the water. Children are totally unpredictable in this respect, and many a small child who is normally into everything, and shows no sign of fear in his everyday activities, will stand on a pool side weeping most piteously at the prospect of going into the water. Much of this can be avoided if the subject of going to the pool for the first time is broached some weeks in advance. The child should be told that all the boys go into one room to undress and all the girls into another – this is very important to some children, and the lack of this information worries them considerably. They should be told that the water is warm, that it is shallow enough for them to stand in. Hearty uncles who want to tell the child that they were taught to swim (usually it happened in the army, according to them) by being thrown into the water at the deep end, should be kept away from the children. One wonders why they say this sort of thing, because invariably it's just not true; but the number of young schoolchildren who go for their first swimming lesson with the suspicion that someone is going to throw or at least put them straight into deep water, makes one wonder about some adults.

Even if you have done all the right things before actually going to the baths, however, it is still possible that the child will display some degree of reluctance actually to get into the water. There is no answer to this other than continual patience, kindness and encouragement. These qualities are easy to display to a child who is emotionally near to you, provided that you do not interpret the situation as being some sort of a reflection on you – and it is very easy to see the situation in this light. ('To think that a child of mine . . .') If you really think about it, the key word in that phrase is 'mine', when it ought to be 'child'. After all, nobody (adult or child) enjoys being in a situation where others see him displaying his fears. The child is not standing there crying, or whatever, just to annoy you, his instincts are to want to please you. He is crying because he's terrified. You know he need not be, and should not be, but he doesn't.

So try to get the child to sit on the side and dangle his feet in the water. Get him to make a big splash with his feet. Get into the water yourself and stand in front of where he is sitting, and when he splashes his feet make a great song and dance about his splashing water into your face. Make him laugh! If this works, try to get him to sit on the top step leading into the pool and do the same. Get him a pair of inflatable armbands to wear, and show him other children wearing them in the water. Be wise enough to recognise the moment when you have got as far with him as you are going to get, and take him out. Tell him how well he splashed his feet in the water, and ask his mother if she saw him splash water in your face so hard that you fell over. Stress how funny it was. All this is so obvious to most parents that there is little need to say it, but a relatively unsuccessful first visit to a swimming pool can put a child off for a long time if his feeling of having let himself down (and young as he might be, he'll probably feel this) is exacerbated by a feeling that he's let you down as well. So be patient, be encouraging, and it will come; it may take some time, but come it will.

Once the child has shown his willingness to go into the water, it is wise to equip him with a flotation aid of some kind, so that, no matter what, he will not sink to the bottom. It is also a great confidence booster. Aids usually available are:

Inflatable armbands. Probably the best aid of them all at this stage. They supply buoyancy in the right place, and are inexpensive to buy. Ensure that replacement stopper-plugs are obtainable before buying.

Inflatable rings. Better than no aid at all, but (except for the highly nervous child, who should wear armbands and a ring) they provide too much buoyancy, and provide it in the wrong place. They inhibit forward movement in the horizontal position and, unless tied on, which is a fiddling business, they slip up and down the trunk and sometimes slip right over the hips, in which case the legs are kept afloat while the head sinks.

Other (worn) inflatables. These come in various shapes and sizes, but none that I have seen are superior to armbands in any respect other than that they cost more.

Inflatables which the child holds, or which are not fixed to the child's body. Avoid these. The child has sufficient problems without having to remember to hold on to an aid.

Aids other than inflatables. These include things like polystyrene floats and flippers which, while invaluable at a later stage, have little benefit at this initial stage.

So, with the child in the water, the following stages must be carefully and patiently tackled:

Getting him to move about freely without the support of the handrail.

Getting his feet off the bottom of the pool.

Submerging the head.

Adopting a horizontal position in the water, and regaining the feet from this position.

Each of these should be fully and confidently achieved by the child before moving on to the next.

Moving about in the water

The following sequence of activities may usefully be used:

1 Walking across the pool, holding the handrail with one hand and your hand with the other.

2 Walking, holding the handrail with both hands.

3 Walking, holding the handrail with one hand.

4 Walking, holding your hand with one hand, with the handrail within grasping distance of the other but not held.

5 Walking, with you walking backwards in front of the child, with your hands outstretched and available to be grasped if necessary.

6 Walking freely. This can be encouraged if you and

the child play with a football-sized plastic ball, throwing it to each other. This will serve two purposes – first, the child will be motivated by the play situation to move toward the ball, and second, when the ball lands near him, it will splash water near to and on to his face, and in this situation he is likely to accept this happily.

Feet off the bottom

1 Facing the pool wall, holding the handrail with both hands; put the child's left foot against the wall.

2 Repeat (1), but lifting the child's right foot to place it against the wall.

3 Same position, but this time put the left foot against the wall, followed by the right foot.

4 See if the child can move along the wall like this, by moving his hands along the rail, and his feet along the wall.

5 Stand the child side-on to the wall, holding the rail with both hands. Encourage the child to lift his feet off the bottom and pull himself along the rail with his hands.

6 Stand facing the child, holding both his hands, and tow him through the water. Do not encourage him to kick his legs about. As you know from the early chapters, this is an exercise in flotation, not propulsion. We want the child to feel the water supporting him, and we do not want him to get the idea that he has to thrash his limbs around in order to float in the horizontal position.

You will notice that at no time in this procedure are you advised to support the child's flotation. No hands under chins, or under tummies, since this is absolutely counter-productive to what you are trying to achieve, which is a confidence in the child that he is able to float in the water. Once you start holding him up, you are convincing him that he can float all the time Daddy, or whoever, is holding him up, and the corollary of this is, 'If Daddy lets go of me, I'll sink'.

Submerging the head

As you know, we are working our way slowly towards the push and glide. In order to do this, we must accustom the child to having his face in the water. All the following exercises are aimed at getting him to accept having his face more or less permanently wet. Therefore he must be discouraged from wiping the water off his face every time it gets wet. It's not natural to have water dripping off the face, but it's very necessary to get used to it.

At some point the child is going to get a mouthful of water, and will probably swallow some. While swallowing water from a swimming pool is not the most attractive experience aesthetically, it will not do any harm. Any unhygienic elements which may have got into the water are rendered safe by the continual purification processes. (This is not true, of course, of untreated water as found in most rivers, lakes and seas.) The unpleasantness of the experience lies in the unexpected way in which it happens; one finds oneself choking and gasping on the amount of water that would normally be drunk in a sip, from a glass. For any learner, this is a frightening experience, and it is particularly so for a child. No one, therefore, is doing a child any favours by telling him that he will not 'get a mouthful', because, at some time or other, he surely will. It is much better to get the child to accept that this might happen, although you take all steps to see that it does not. When you are playing with him, throwing balls, splashing each other, tell him from time to time that you just swallowed a mouthful, but as a matter of interest, not as a matter of alarm. Try to get the message across to him that this is normal, not abnormal.

When water unexpectedly enters your mouth, there are but two choices open to you. Either swallow it, or spit it out! Both are easy, natural actions and neither is harmful. Both may be aesthetically unpleasant, but not harmful; when you do neither, but, as a panic reflex, you inhale some of it, this can be a most unpleasant experience. We owe it to the child to train him to accept as normal the presence of water around and sometimes in his mouth, so that the panic reflex does not happen. I have always made a point of telling children that during the course of learning to swim they'll probably swallow a pint of pool water and that every time they swallow some leaves them that much less to swallow before they've completed the pint. I say this in a very light-hearted way, but it seems to work with most of them, since they make a point of proudly announcing the fact, every time they get a mouthful – and most of the time they are spitting it out!

Messing about with a ball is a good starting point. Encourage the child to make the ball splash your face, and make a great fuss about it. Make him laugh. You must, of course, be very gentle with him at first, but he will soon get used to more and more splashing.

77

Let this lead on to deliberately splashing one another with the hands.

Crouch down in the water, take a deep breath and close your lips. Then crouch a bit lower, so that the water is at mouth level, and make a forcible 'Brrrrrrrrrr' sound with your lips. This produces a very funny high-pitched bubbling sound which children seem to find absolutely hilarious. If you can learn to do this yourself, and get the child to copy you, he will get so engrossed in trying to produce this sound that he will not realise that in the course of doing it he is taking water into his mouth and ejecting it. As far as one can be accurate in a matter like this, the air should be expelled at about one eighth of an inch below the surface to produce this sound, which sounds rather like a demented Donald Duck!

Any other play activities where the child will be getting water on his face and head, can be used to advantage. You can ask him to blow bubbles into the water, which he can practise in a hand basin at home. In my experience it does not work to ask a child, at this stage, merely to stand there and put his head under the water for no reason other than the doing of it. If he gets his head under in the course of doing something pleasurable,

he's likely to accept it as all part of the game, but he is likely to reject the cold-blooded approach because he has to make a conscious effort to do it.

Adopting a horizontal position in the water

This should start with towing the child. Face him, hold both his hands, and walk slowly backwards. Your hands, and thus the child's hands, should be in the water. If you hold his hands above the water, the laws of flotation will make it impossible for him to achieve a horizontal posture. You should ask the child to make his arms long. His immediate reaction to being towed will probably be to bend his arms so that he can lever himself upward and bring his head and shoulders clear of the water. In other words, he will be inclined to use your arms as a platform which he can use to lift himself up and out of the water. With arms fully extended, he will use your hands properly, as a support which he really does not need, but which he does not yet realise he does not need. Before you start, tell him to take a deep breath and to close his lips tightly. Later on you can ask the child to lower his head so that his face is in the water.

Regaining the feet from the horizontal position is best

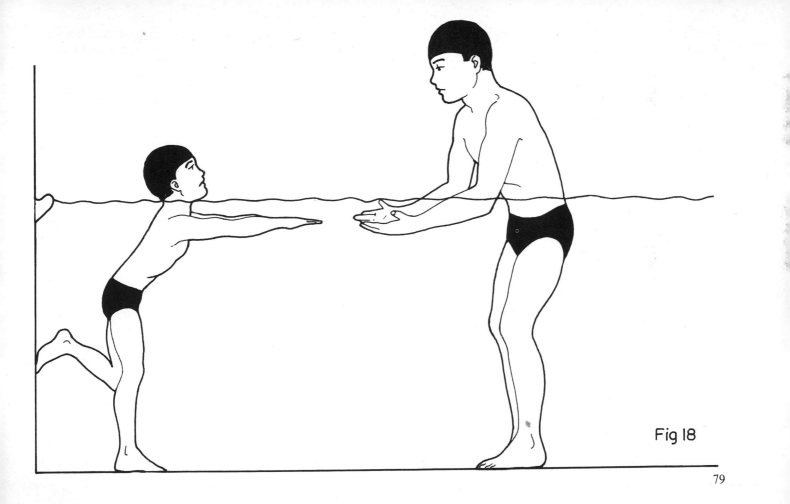

Fig 18

initiated from towing, since you are in a position to assist the child to regain his feet by a little judicious lifting. The procedure is as outlined in Chapter 2, and as illustrated in Fig 3.

Tow the child on his back. Stand behind him with your hands under his armpits. Ask him to lie back on the water as you walk slowly backwards. It is important that the child puts his head back on to the water, so that his ears are just clear of the surface. Teach regaining the feet as outlined in Chapter 2.

Stand the child with his back to the pool wall. Stand facing him, with your arms stretched out towards him, with your hands just below the surface and about three feet from his hands. Ask him to push himself toward you and grasp your hands. (*See Fig 18.*) This is a rudimentary push and glide, so it is important that the child starts with arms outstretched and shoulders under the water.

Gradually increase the distance over which the child glides, but let him be the arbiter of the distance. Do not push him. Having got so far, it is important not to frighten him just when you are at the point where he is nearly ready to be taught to swim.

Let the child stand three or four feet from the wall, facing it, and push and glide to the handrail. You should stand beside him, but only to grab him should anything go wrong. Do not try, or offer, to support him in any way.

Finally, let him start from the wall and push and glide outward and regain the standing position at the end of the glide.

Somewhere along this line of events, the child should be persuaded to abandon his flotation aid and to substitute a polystyrene float. Only the person who is teaching him can know when the right moment has arrived, but the time to start thinking about it is when he starts on this final group of activities. From here on, the confidence exercises he will need to do are the same as were outlined in Chapter 2, excluding those which would take him out of his depth. Once he is doing a competent and confident push and glide, he is ready to be taught to swim, and to swim well!

Which stroke first?

It really does not matter which stroke is taught first. Some children show an obvious preference for swimming on the back in the initial stages, and these children should be taught Back Crawl as a first stroke. Those who seem happier on the front could be started on either Crawl or Breast Stroke. You should get some indication of which would be better for the child by watching his legs when he is being towed, or when he is playing about with push and glide and similar activities. If his legs tend to move in an up-and-down pattern, then start him on Crawl. If he attempts a frog-like kick, then Breast Stroke should be his first stroke.

Whichever stroke it is to be, the procedures are exactly as outlined in the preceding chapters on stroke technique, but do remember that children tend to learn more easily if they can see a demonstration of what they are to try to do. They tend to copy movements, since they are unable to rationalise and analyse in the way most adults are able to do.

In any public swimming pool, there is always someone swimming a stroke well enough for you to be able to point out to the child what it is you want him to do. People who swim a stroke reasonably well are almost invariably flattered if someone asks them if they would do a slow length so that a child may be shown the way to swim the stroke properly, and they will usually be pleased to do so. Just one point – if your pool is one in which competitive swimmers train during public sessions, do not break into someone's training schedule to make this request. Do wait until he has finished.

A child needs to be shown the full stroke, so that he may gain insight into what he is eventually aiming at. Having seen this, he needs his attention specifically drawn to that part of the stroke that he is going to practise. Having watched someone swimming Crawl, for example, he should be told, 'Now watch those legs – see how nice and straight they are?', before he goes to practise the leg action, with you continually reminding him that he should keep his legs straight.

Having got the child to this point, the best thing to do is to make him a member of the local swimming club. And while you are at it, why not join yourself?

12　Resuscitation

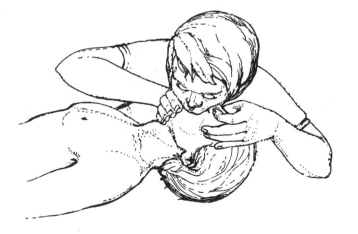

I could not conclude a book on swimming without mentioning that which I consider to be the responsibility of all of us – the responsibility to save life. Quite obviously, the more people who learn to swim, the smaller will be the number who drown, although the simple ability to swim, if defined as 'being able to propel oneself through water without support', will not always prevent a person from drowning. This is why I make such a point of complete water confidence as a necessary pre-requisite to the actual techniques of swimming. Many people who were able to swim a little have drowned because they suddenly found themselves in the water in an unfamiliar position. In that unfamiliar position, probably in the grip of growing panic, they have been unable to assume a posture in which they were able to swim. The same thing happens regularly to people who are able to swim a bit, but who find themselves in the water fully clothed and do not know how to cope, particularly if they happen to be wearing gumboots which immediately fill with water.

The ability to cope with situations of this kind can be fairly simply gained by the acquisition of swimming survival skills, as exemplified in the Amateur Swimming Association's various survival schemes. Any swimming pool manager or local swimming club would be pleased to give you the details.

While it is obviously desirable for people to be able to swim enough to keep themselves out of trouble in water and, ideally, to be able to drag out those who are unable to keep themselves out of trouble, it is still probable that there will always be times when people need help as the result of accidents in water, and it is possible that any one of us might be the one whose action, or lack of it, might mean the difference between life or death for some poor unfortunate. Even if we are unable to render assistance to someone who is in trouble in the water, we should all be able to do the right thing when, by some means or other, the victim is pulled out. Quite often the person who effected the actual rescue, having got the victim to dry land, is too exhausted to be able to undertake the next step, and must at this point look to an onlooker to take over.

We have to assume that anyone who is pulled out of water unconscious is probably dying, and will die unless someone does the right thing, and does it quickly. The right thing to do, unless there are most unusual complications in the form of severe facial injuries, is to apply what has come to be called 'the kiss of life' or, to give it its correct title, resuscitation by the expired air method.

This is what to do, as quickly as possible:

1   Put the patient on his back.

2   Tilt his head back so that his chin is pointing upward.

3   Pull his lower jaw down so that his mouth opens, and run your forefinger around the inside of his mouth and throat to ensure that there is nothing in there which could block the air passage. If there is, hook it out. With the patient's mouth open, pinch his nostrils firmly between the thumb and forefinger.

5   Cover the patient's mouth with your own and blow into it, four times, at the rate of one blow per second, watching his chest as you do so. His chest will rise.

6 Remove your mouth from his, and watch his chest fall. Then resume blowing into his mouth once every five seconds, removing your mouth between blowing actions.

7 Watch the rise and fall of the patient's chest all the time. What you are doing is only potentially effective if the patient's chest is rising as you blow air into him and falling as you remove your mouth.

This procedure may be carried out by holding the patient's mouth in a tightly closed position and blowing into his nose – both methods are equally effective. The important thing, from the viewpoint of the poor unfortunate lying there, is that somebody does one of them, and quickly! He will not want to argue about which method you used when he regains consciousness.

One last word. This is not always a very pleasant thing to have to do. Most people have an aesthetic revulsion to putting their mouth to the mouth of someone they do not know. Accept the fact, now, that it probably will not be a pleasant task, and if the time comes, get in there and do it just the same.

Appendix A

Addresses

Amateur Swimming Association
Harold Fern House
Derby Square
Loughborough
Leicestershire LE11 OAL

Royal Life Saving Society
14 Devonshire Street
London W1

Scottish Amateur Swimming Association
16 Royal Crescent
Glasgow G3 7SL

Swimming Teachers Association*
Queens College Chambers
38a Paradise Street
Birmingham 1

Welsh Amateur Swimming Association
45 Devon Place
Newport

*Also promotes personal performance and teaching award schemes.

Sports Council
The Sports Council
70 Brompton Road
London SW3 1EX
Tel: 01-589 3411

REGIONAL OFFICES
The Sports Council
Northern Region
*Northumberland, Cumbria, Durham, Cleveland and
Metropolitan County of Tyne and Wear*
County Court Building
9 Hallgarth Street
Durham DH1 3PB
Tel: 0385 64278/9

The Sports Council
North West Region
*Lancashire, Cheshire, Greater Manchester
and Merseyside*
Byrom House
Quay Street
Manchester M3 5FJ
Tel: 061 834 9573/0338

The Sports Council
Yorkshire and Humberside Region
*W. Yorkshire, S. Yorkshire, N. Yorkshire
and Humberside*
5 St Paul's Street
Leeds LS1 2NQ
Tel: 0532 36443/4

The Sports Council
East Midland Region
*Derbyshire, Nottinghamshire, Lincolnshire,
Leicestershire and Northamptonshire*
26 Musters Road
West Bridgford
Nottingham NG2 7PL
Tel: 0602 861325/6

The Sports Council
West Midlands Region
*Metropolitan County, Hereford, Worcester, Salop,
Staffordshire and Warwickshire*
Crest House
7 Highfield Road
Edgbaston
Birmingham B15 3EG
Tel: 021 454 3808/9

The Sports Council
Eastern Region
Norfolk, Cambridgeshire, Suffolk, Bedfordshire, Hertfordshire and Essex
26–28 Bromham Road
Bedford MK40 2QD
Tel: 0234 44281

The Sports Council
Greater London and South East Region
Greater London, Surrey, Kent, and East and West Sussex
160 Great Portland Street
London W1N 5TB
Tel: 01-580 9092/7

The Sports Council
Southern Region
Hampshire, Isle of Wight, Berkshire, Buckinghamshire and Oxfordshire
Watlington House
Watlington Street
Reading RG1 4RJ
Berkshire
Tel: 0734 52342/57740

The Sports Council
South Western Region
Avon, Cornwall, Devon, Dorset, Somerset, Wiltshire and Gloucestershire
Ashlands House
Ashlands
Crewkerne
Somerset TA18 7LQ
Tel: 0460 31 3491

Appendix B

Award Schemes for the Non-competitive Swimmer promoted by the Amateur Swimming Association:

1   Personal Survival Awards
at three progressive levels, ie bronze, silver and gold. Designed to promote, test and reward the ability to survive in water. Deal with swimming and general watermanship skills needed in emergency situations. Interesting and fun to do.

2   The Million Scheme
by registering as a member of this scheme and logging your swims, you can become a member of the ASA Million Club – a daunting thought when you start, but it adds something to your training sessions.

Details of these schemes, and others may be obtained from your local baths Manager, the local swimming club, the Sports Council – local or regional (see addresses on page 85).

Further Reading

Amateur Swimming Association. *Better Swimming* (EP Sports Series).
——. *Survival Swimming* (EP Sports Series).
——. *The Teaching of Swimming* (Obtainable from bookshops or directly from the ASA).
John M. Hogg. *Learning to Swim* (EP Sports Series).

Acknowledgements

During the time that I have spent writing this book, I have become increasingly aware of the fact that my philosophy and techniques of teaching swimming are an amalgam of the knowledge that I have acquired from others, over a long period of years. I would, therefore, wish to take this opportunity of acknowledging my indebtedness to John Lewis, sometime PE Organiser of the Borough of Blackpool, who, when I was a young teacher made me take the first transitional step from swimmer to teacher by taking me through the course leading to the ASA Teachers' Certificate for Swimming; to Mike Melanefy, HMI, who took me through the course for the Advanced Teachers' Certificate; to W. Mc. D. (Don) Cameron, who guided my first steps as an examiner for the ASA and later taught me how to tutor a course; to Alan Donlan, Dick Underwood, Jackie Brayshaw, Tom Saunders and other colleagues on ASA sub-committees, from whom I have learned a great deal in discussions; to the many people who have attended my courses to learn to swim, or to learn to teach swimming, and by their reactions have enabled me to evaluate the procedures I have advocated. My thanks go especially to my friend and colleague, Brian Clayton, an archetypal 'stubborn non-swimmer'. During the many, many hours we spent together in the water, his scientific mind was able to assess, from the learner's point of view, the strengths and weaknesses of the various practices that I put him through. Although he now enjoys his swimming, I probably learned more than he did. To all these poeple, my affectionate gratitude. I would also wish to acknowledge the efforts of Bob Hogarth, who produced the delightful art work

from references which mainly consisted of badly drawn pin men; of Joyce Braithwaite, who produces perfect typescript from very poor originals in record time, and above all, of my wife, who reads, corrects, suggests, or encourages and generally keeps me going.
J.K.L.
September 1975

Index